Medical Analogies for Clinician-Patient Communication

Muhammad Azaan Khan
Gizem Ashraf • Hamza Ashraf
Editors

Medical Analogies for Clinician-Patient Communication

Innovative Strategies for Improving the Clinical Encounter

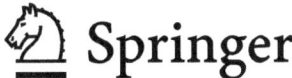 Springer

Editors
Muhammad Azaan Khan
University of New South Wales
Sydney, NSW, Australia

Gizem Ashraf
Monash University
Monash Health
Melbourne, VIC, Australia

Hamza Ashraf
Monash University
Austin Health
Melbourne, VIC, Australia

ISBN 978-3-030-87292-2   ISBN 978-3-030-87293-9   (eBook)
https://doi.org/10.1007/978-3-030-87293-9

This Springer imprint is published by the registered company Springer Nature
Switzerland AG
The registered company address is: Gewerbestrasse 11, 6330 Cham, Switzerland

Foreword

From the standpoint of medicine as art for the prevention and cure of disease, the man who translates the hieroglyphics of science into the plain language of healing is certainly the most useful. – Sir William Osler

Communication is the key to the success of any societal interaction. Perhaps nowhere is this truer than in healthcare, where the quality of this interaction is the basis for all that follows. Quite simply, if the doctor-patient communication is compromised, then so too is the health outcome, and there is a mounting body of research confirming this (Ha).

One of the biggest barriers to effective communication is, ironically, a result of the very historical and scientific basis of our profession. Jargon. As medical students, we are taught about anatomy, physiology and pathology using unfamiliar words with ancient Greek or Latin origins. Once we begin work as junior doctors, this is then couched in an equally bewildering array of technical terminology about clinical tests, drugs and procedures. Sir William Osler's description of the 'hieroglyphics of science' is spot on.

All of which is hard enough for this select group of highly intelligent, educated and motivated people having to learn this 'language of medicine' – our university and college students. Imagine how difficult it must be then for our poor patients to understand us?

The concept of health literacy is central to addressing this gulf. It is defined as "the degree to which individuals have the capacity to obtain, process, and understand basic health information and services needed to make appropriate health decisions" (Nielsen). Remember that you, dear reader, are by definition privileged with high health literacy (otherwise you wouldn't be interested in this book!). Most of our patients are, however, not, and have low health literacy. Especially those for whom we worry about the most – the socially, culturally and economically disadvantaged (Graham).

Exacerbating the problem is the fact that we aren't nearly as clever as we think we are. Research has confirmed that in our conversations with patients and their carers, our perceptions of their understanding is vastly different to theirs. One study into surgical consultations found that almost 75% of the doctors rated their communication as satisfactory, compared to only 20% of their patients! (Tongue).

One factor behind this is our inherent, automatic tendency to speak in scientific 'medical' English. 'Jargon-oblivion' is a term coined recently that refers to this 'discrepancy between our self-rated skill in clear communication and our patients' ability to understand the terms we use' (Pitt). So you can see that awareness itself is a starting point to becoming better communicators.

Changing the way we speak to our patients is critical if we want to ensure they have the best possible chance of getting better. Our dazzling clinical skills will amount to little if they are not matched with competent communication skills.

Which is what this excellent book is all about.

Even after just a few years' experience, the authors have realised the importance of the need to speak more clearly and simply to patients and their carers. It's not just 'what' we say that matters, but equally 'how' we say it.

The solution presented in this book is a deceptively simple one – analogies that derive from everyday experiences and are therefore much more likely to be understood. Language free of jargon, thereby avoiding 'medical' English and using common terms instead.

This in fact is what we end up doing subconsciously after spending time in clinical settings. It makes sense then that educators can help accelerate the process by showing how to communicate more effectively from the earliest stages of training. What you are holding in your hands is a clever yet endearing way to help achieve this competency.

I look forward to trying out these analogies in the clinic, wards and lecture theatres, and have already learnt some useful ones I hadn't come across! I commend the authors for taking the time and effort to put themselves in the patient's shoes and see the world from the other side of the consultation.

Perhaps then we can, together, start deciphering the *hieroglyphics* of medicine and make our vocation truly patient friendly.

Ashish Agar
University of New South Wales
Sydney, NSW, Australia

References

1. Ha JF, Longnecker N. Doctor-patient communication: a review. Ochsner J. 2010;20;10(1):38–43.
2. Nielsen-Bohlman L, Panzer AM, Kindig DA, editors. Health literacy: a prescription to end confusion. Washington, DC: National Academies Press; 2004.
3. Graham S, Brookey J. Do patients understand? Perm J. 2008;12(3):67–9.
4. Tongue JR, Epps HR, Forese LL. Communication skills for patient-centered care: research-based, easily learned techniques for medical interviews that benefit orthopaedic surgeons and their patients. J Bone Joint Surg Am. 2005; 87:652–8.
5. Pitt MB, Hendrickson MA. Eradicating Jargon-Oblivion—a proposed classification system of medical Jargon. J Gen Intern Med. 2019;35(6):1861–4.

Preface

The seedling for this book sprouted from a conversation between a surgeon and a patient. In a few meagre minutes, an elderly patient was awoken, informed that they had fractured their hip and would be operated on in a few hours, told to fast until then, and the upcoming procedure explained. Despite the surgeon's best efforts to minimise medical jargon, the look of confusion on the patient's face belied a less-than-ideal understanding of what was happening to them. This isn't an isolated scenario, but unfortunately one that many of us have likely experienced. The reasons why are valid, but they don't legitimise how unbalancing and disempowering these brisk conversations are to patient-centred care.

Clearly, there is need for an efficient way to translate years of study and experiential learning from the doctor and healthcare professional to the patient. The best vehicle for doing this, we found, is through analogies with our shared experiences, our humanity.

From that simple seedling, we created a reference book which provides analogies for many of the medical conditions we commonly encounter. After much time from the authors creating and pruning analogies, we hope that this book can serve as a fruitful reference for anyone wanting to communicate profoundly with their patients without forfeiting brevity.

As doctors and healthcare professionals, we are fortunate to learn by standing on the shoulders of giants. We hope that this book helps us elevate patients to similar heights.

Sydney, NSW, Australia	Muhammad Azaan Khan
Melbourne, VIC, Australia	Gizem Ashraf
Melbourne, VIC, Australia	Hamza Ashraf

Acknowledgement

Firstly, we would like to thank our seniors and mentors for all the wisdom they have distilled for us from years and decades of service. Their words are a guiding light for times of uncertainty, and a priceless map to understanding the patient and having them understand us. Credit must also be given to our peers whose contributions have rounded this book, particularly Niyaz Mostafa, Samed Onder, Ali Abid, Tajrian Amin, Moudrack Sjarief, Adil Lathif, Mohamed Ismail, Mohammad Alwahwah, and Syed Ali Ahsan. Finally, we must thank the people who privilege and enrich our lives the most, our patients.

Sydney, NSW, Australia	Muhammad Azaan Khan
Melbourne, VIC, Australia	Gizem Ashraf
Melbourne, VIC, Australia	Hamza Ashraf

Contents

Contributors

Muhammad Azaan Khan University of New South Wales, Sydney, NSW, Australia

Gizem Ashraf Monash Health, Monash University, Melbourne, VIC, Australia

Hamza Ashraf Austin Health, Monash University, Melbourne, VIC, Australia

Imaan Ashraf James Cook University, Douglas, QLD, Australia

Saad Ashraf Monash University, Clayton, VIC, Australia

Zehra Hasimoglu Latrobe University, Melbourne, VIC, Australia

Yusuf Hassan The University of Melbourne, Melbourne, VIC, Australia

Alisha Rawal Monash University, Clayton, VIC, Australia

Qazi Sarem Shahab University of New South Wales, Sydney, NSW, Australia

Cardiology

1

Muhammad Azaan Khan, Gizem Ashraf,
Hamza Ashraf, Saad Ashraf,
Yusuf Hassan, Alisha Rawal,
Imaan Ashraf, Qazi Sarem Shahab,
and Zehra Hasimoglu

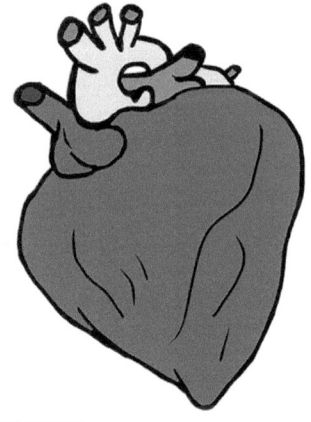

M. A. Khan (✉) · Q. S. Shahab
University of New South Wales, Sydney, NSW, Australia

G. Ashraf
Monash Health, Monash University, Melbourne, VIC, Australia

H. Ashraf
Austin Health, Monash University, Melbourne, VIC, Australia

S. Ashraf · A. Rawal
Monash University, Clayton, VIC, Australia

Y. Hassan
The University of Melbourne, Melbourne, VIC, Australia

I. Ashraf
James Cook University, Douglas, QLD, Australia

Z. Hasimoglu
Latrobe University, Melbourne, VIC, Australia

Contents

Angina

Car Running Out of Fuel

Experiencing chest pain can be compared to rusty fuel supply pipes in the engine of an old car. A car needs well-maintained fuel pipes to keep its engine running. Similarly, your heart needs functioning arteries which deliver blood to your heart. In times of added blood demand, your heart makes a cry for help because it isn't getting enough blood through its clogged pipes. This cry for help manifests as severe chest pain and tells the body to rest to reduce the demand on the heart. This is also a warning sign that the pipes or arteries need to be cleaned to prevent another serious blockage.

Aneurysm

Water Balloon

Usually, your blood vessels are sturdy like a hose full of water, but sometimes there is a weakness along the wall, which causes a bulge to occur. We call this bulge an aneurysm. Aneurysms are like water balloons. As the water is travelling through the hose, the bulging water balloon allows for some pooling of the water. However, the water balloon can only handle a certain amount of pressure before it stops stretching and bursts. Similarly, an aneurysm has the risk of rupturing if the pressure of the blood inside it becomes too great.

Aortic Dissection

Earthquake

An aortic dissection is a tear in your aorta, which can be compared to an earthquake fault line, which is a tear in the earth. Initially, an invisible fault line develops underneath the ground which we cannot see. This is like the invisible tear which develops in the aorta but does not cause any symptoms initially. Eventually, the fault line gets so bad that an earthquake occurs. Similarly, the invisible tear in the aorta gets large enough to cause that region of the aorta to dissect. Just as an earthquake can have aftershocks some time afterwards, a dissection can also progress further in size which can lead to life-threatening haemorrhage.

Arrhythmias

Orchestra Conductor

Usually, the heart beats in a steady rhythm, like it is being directed by the conductor of an orchestra. However, sometimes the conductor changes the rhythm. For example, the conductor might start conducting faster and so your heart rate speeds up. At other times, your heart rhythm might change. This is like the conductor missing a beat or going off the script.

Air Traffic Controller and Hackers

The air traffic controller is in charge of making sure that airplanes enter and leave the airport in an organised manner without crashing into each other. If the air traffic control system was hacked and started sending out random signals, there would be nothing but chaos, and planes might crash into each other. There would be haphazard plane traffic at the airport as there would be lack of direction.

The planes are like the blood in our heart and the air traffic controller is like the electrical node, which is a specific area designed to control the rate of the impulses that allow the heart to beat. Usually, the node functions normally and directs the blood flow in an organised fashion. However, this area can be 'hacked' or overtaken by other aberrant cells which start sending random signals to the entire heart. The beating of the heart, and therefore the blood flow control, is no longer organized. Just like there was a traffic jam with the planes, there can be a traffic jam in the heart which causes a blood clot.

Atherosclerosis

Volcano

Think of an atherosclerotic plaque in your blood vessels like a volcano. Initially, the volcano lays dormant and doesn't pose a threat. Over time the pressure keeps building up and the volcano fills with lava. This is like the atherosclerotic plaque filling with cholesterol and undergoing further inflammation. Eventually, the pressure in the volcano increases to an extent that the cap of the volcano bursts and the lava spills out. A similar process happens to atherosclerotic plaques. The ruptured contents from the plaque can block downstream arteries in any organ.

Cardiac Arrest

Power Outage

We can think of your heart as an electrical appliance and the arteries supplying blood to it as electrical wires. If one of the wires supplying an appliance is damaged, the appliance ceases to function. Similarly, in a cardiac arrest, if one of the arteries supplying the heart gets blocked, the heart can lose its ability to pump the blood efficiently around the body.

Cardiomyopathy

Bicycle with Motorcycle Wheels

In patients with cardiomyopathy, the muscular walls of the heart are thicker than usual. This is similar to wheels for bicycles and motorcycles. Riding a bicycle with thin bicycle wheels is quite easy but if someone was to replace the wheels of your bicycle with motorcycle tyres, you would struggle to pedal. In cardiomyopathy, the muscles are thickened like a motorbike tyre, meaning the heart needs to exert a greater force to pump blood.

Congestive Heart failure – Pathophysiology

Faulty Balloon Pump

A balloon can be used as an air pump, by inflating it with air and then releasing that air rapidly. Imagine your heart as one of these balloon air pumps. However, this pump can fail.

Firstly, if the walls of the balloon thicken and stiffen over time, the balloon can no longer stretch to increase capacity; thus, the balloon can no longer fill with enough air. Similarly, a heart with thickened walls can no longer fill with blood, resulting in less blood being pumped around the body. This is called diastolic heart failure.

Alternatively, the balloon air pump may have been over-stretched over the years by constantly being filled with too much air. If the walls have been overstretched, they can lose their elasticity. Elasticity is what makes a full balloon push out all its air and deflate rapidly when you release your grip on it. Similarly, when the heart loses its elasticity, it can no longer pump blood effectively. This is called systolic heart failure.

Congestive Heart Failure – Treatment

Horse Pulling Sandbags

In congestive heart failure, your heart is working very hard but inefficiently, like a tired horse pulling a cart full of sandbags. One of the ways to help the horse is to reduce the number of sandbags on the cart, thus reducing its workload. For this, we can reduce the fluid overload in the body which will control the amount of blood going into your heart. Once this is achieved, your heart will be less exhausted, enabling it to pump more efficiently.

Alternatively, you can encourage the horse to work harder by dangling a carrot in front of it. Similarly, we can give medications that stimulate the heart to work harder when it is tiring.

Another way we can use to ensure our horse isn't tired all the time is to control its pace, maintaining a steady, moderate pumping rate. This is achieved by either inserting a pacemaker into the heart or using medications to control the pace of the heart and prevent over-exhaustion of its muscles.

Deep Vein Thrombosis (DVT) and Pulmonary Embolus (PE)

Blocked River

Imagine your bloodstream as a river that branches off into many different other streams and creeks. Over the years, a riverbank accumulates various types of debris: rocks, tree bark, logs, etc. Occasionally, some of this debris can break off the riverbank, enter the river and lodge downstream, thus blocking the river flow and depriving everyone downstream of vital water supply.

Similarly, the walls of your blood vessels also have debris, particularly fat deposits, and these can break off in a similar fashion, block off downstream blood supply and deprive downstream organs of vital blood supply for sustaining their function. This particular example is called a thromboembolic event. When this happens in your brain, it's called an embolic stroke. This can happen in your lungs too and would be termed a pulmonary embolism.

Rotten Milk

A DVT is when you have a clot in one of your deep leg veins. Your blood that has clotted is like mlik that has thickened and curdled. Imagine trying to pour the milk. As you keep pouring, eventually the curds at the bottom will go to the mouth of the bottle and get stuck, so you can't pour any more. This can happen to block the vessels supplying your lungs, cutting off the supply to them. To keep allowing flow, we need to remove the curd, or in your case, the clot. We either do this by breaking it up using medication or manually removing it. Then, we need to find out why the milk is going bad and thickening to form curds, which means finding out why your blood is thickening easily and forming clots.

Hyperlipidaemia

Bakery

Within a bakery, you have your basic ingredients, machines to make bread and eventually when your bread goes bad or there's too much of it on the shelf, a cleaner to remove the excess bread. The cholesterol in your body is managed in a similar production line.

Just as some bread in your diet is necessary, so too is a moderate level of cholesterol for bodily functions. However, things go bad when the production line of cholesterol produces too much, or produces the two different types of cholesterol in the wrong ratios.

There are two types of cholesterol. The LDL cholesterol is like an untidy teenager who goes around the house dropping things anywhere and everywhere. HDL cholesterol is like a house proud mum who goes around putting things at their right place. Higher levels of LDL and lower levels of HDL predispose people to developing cardiovascular disease.

Considering our bakery example, one way to produce too much bread is to have more basic ingredients available. More flour and yeast equals more bread. Similarly, more cholesterol in your diet can lead to more cholesterol in your body.

Another way to have more bread on the shelf is to have machines that go into overdrive and produce undesirable, large amounts. Similarly, some people are born with overactive mechanisms to produce large amounts of LDL cholesterol.

Finally, if the bakery doesn't have a cleaner to remove all the bad bread from the shelf, over time the store will become overrun with bread. Similarly, if the body doesn't have enough HDL cholesterol, then the LDL cholesterol can increase.

Hypertension

Water Network

Your circulatory system is like the local water network. If the pressure within the water system becomes elevated, some of the pipes are likely to burst. The smallest and weakest pipes are more likely to burst. Relating this to the body, high pressures within the blood vessels would put the weakest or smallest vessels at risk of bursting. These smallest blood vessels are in the brain, the kidneys, the eyes, and in the heart. If the burst occurred in the brain, that would be a stroke. In the kidneys and eyes, the high pressures will cause slow damage over time. Unfortunately, the damage happens so slowly that you only notice it when too much damage has been done.

Ischaemic Heart Disease (IHD)

Clogged Pipes

Think of the blood vessels to your heart as narrow pipes. When you're young, these pipes are clean, new and allow perfect blood flow. Old age, smoking and poor diet can cause gunk and rust to gather on the pipe walls. Consequently, the blood can't get through the pipes as smoothly, resulting in reduced blood flow to the heart.

Lymphoedema

Blocked Roof Gutter Drains

Think of your veins as roof gutters and your lymphatic system as its drainage system. Whenever there is excess fluid in your veins, the lymphatics drains it seamlessly. However, if the drainage system gets blocked, the roof gutters overflow, and the water spills over the side onto your house. This is similar to the blockage of the lymph drainage system, so the extra fluid spills out of your lymph vessels and causes you to have swelling in your hands and legs. This phenomenon is known as lymphoedema.

Pericardial Tamponade

Suffocated Heart

Your heart exists in a protective sac with space around it to expand freely. However, if there is a leak into the heart's sac and it fills too much with any kind of fluid, the heart becomes suffocated with no space to expand. If your heart can't expand, it can't fill with enough blood to pump to the rest of your body.

Peripheral Vascular Disease (PVD)

Jammed Windows in the House

This disease can be explained using the example of closed windows on a hot summer day. To be able to handle the soaring temperature on a hot day, you need as many windows as possible to be opened in the house on that day. Think of your blood vessels to your legs and feet as those windows. When you're young, these vessels are open wide and blood flow is perfectly fine. Just as gunk and rust can build up on the window frame, old age, smoking and poor diet can cause gunk to gather on the vessel walls. Consequently, the blood can't get through the vessels smoothly, resulting in less blood flow to your lower limbs. In times of added blood demand, like when you walk, your leg muscles make a cry for help through pain because they aren't getting enough blood through the vessels that are barely patent.

Valvular Heart Disease

Rusty Door

Your heart has four chambers, which can be thought of as rooms in a house. There is a door between each room, which can be thought as the valves in the heart. When the house is new, the doors work normally and open without any issue. However, over time rust can build up in the hinges of the doors, which makes it more difficult for them to open and they can even get stuck. Similarly, the valves can get damaged over time, which makes it more difficult for them to open. Just like we can hear a rusty door creaking as it opens, we can hear a murmur as the blood flows through the damaged valve.

Varicose Veins – Pathology

Interstate Highway

Our body's venous system can be compared to multiple roads merging to converge onto a highway. The deep venous system is the interstate highway, the superficial system is a series of multiple, less wide roads.

Blood clots in the superficial system, although painful and troublesome, are usually not a hazard to health. The obstructing clot shunts blood into the deep system, traffic flows without an issue.

In contrast, clots in the deep system are similar to blockages in the interstate highway. When the interstate highway is blocked, travel is re-routed to secondary roads (the superficial system), which have great trouble coping with this burden; traffic is backed up for kilometres. Pressure in the leg veins rises making them tortuous. The extremities swell with fluid (oedema), and blood flow diminishes to a crawl. This is what happens in varicose veins.

Varicose Veins – Treatment

River

Varicose veins are caused by blood backing up into the veins in your legs. We can think of this like a big river feeding into smaller rivers downstream. The big river is the main vein in the leg, and the smaller rivers are the varicose veins we can see. If we build a dam to block each individual small river without actually blocking the larger main river, we may stop the smaller rivers temporarily but eventually the larger river will just produce more smaller rivers elsewhere. This is like treating the varicose veins without treating the main vein – we may have temporary relief but the recurrence rate will be high.

We need to build a dam which blocks the larger river first, and the smaller rivers will just dry off by themselves. If any smaller rivers remain, then we can just build smaller dams to block them off later. Similarly, if we treat the main vein in the leg which is causing the issue, then this will automatically cause the smaller varicose veins to dry up. If any are left, we can go in and treat them directly.

Dermatology

Muhammad Azaan Khan, Gizem Ashraf,
Hamza Ashraf, Saad Ashraf,
Yusuf Hassan, Alisha Rawal,
Imaan Ashraf, Qazi Sarem Shahab,
and Zehra Hasimoglu

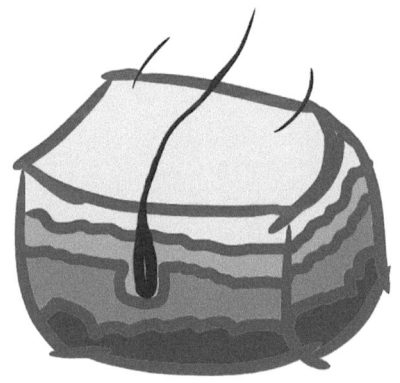

M. A. Khan (✉) · Q. S. Shahab
University of New South Wales, Sydney, NSW, Australia

G. Ashraf
Monash Health, Monash University, Melbourne, VIC, Australia

H. Ashraf
Austin Health, Monash University, Melbourne, VIC, Australia

© The Author(s), under exclusive license to Springer Nature
Switzerland AG 2022
M. A. Khan et al. (eds.), *Medical Analogies for Clinician-Patient
Communication*, https://doi.org/10.1007/978-3-030-87293-9_2

13

S. Ashraf · A. Rawal
Monash University, Clayton, VIC, Australia

Y. Hassan
The University of Melbourne, Melbourne, VIC, Australia

I. Ashraf
James Cook University, Douglas, QLD, Australia

Z. Hasimoglu
Latrobe University, Melbourne, VIC, Australia

Contents

Acne

Infected Caves Within a Mountain Face

Your skin is like a mountain face with little caves. These caves can get clogged up and filled with bacteria, which can cause infection. To treat them, we need to restructure the mountain face to ensure no caves remain, thus there is no space for recurring infections to nest. This restructuring can take a while, and this is why acne treatment can take a long time.

Actinic Keratosis

Cracked Car Paint

Actinic keratosis is like a car that has been in the sun for an extremely long time. After a while parts of the paint on the car will start to crack and peel and flake away. Similarly, after prolonged sun exposure, actinic keratosis can occur and can present as flaky and crusty skin. However, the difference is, the skin decides to continue to grow abnormally and can become malignant.

Collagen

Foundation of a House

Collagen in your skin is like the foundation of a house, which provides the structural support. If the foundation is damaged, you can get cracks in the walls of a house. Similarly, if the collagen in your skin is damaged, then you can have damaged skin which will look scarred. We can fix this by breaking up the old collagen with laser treatment so it can grow and become healthy gain.

Collagen and Elastin

Scaffolding and Springs

Collagen and elastin are proteins in your skin, the amount of which reduces as we age. Collagen is like scaffolding that gives skin its structure – when the scaffolding breaks down, we get wrinkles. Elastin is like a spring which keeps our skin elastic – when elastin is reduced, our skin loses its ability to bounce back and starts to sag.

Cyst

Water Balloon

A cyst is like a balloon with water in it.

Herpes Warts

Spy

The herpes virus can live in the body undetected for years because it is like a spy which puts on a disguise and acts like a friend to hide in our ranks. Our body's immune system doesn't recognise the disguise and therefore doesn't fight it off. It is only after the disguise is taken off many years later that the virus is revealed to the body and the immune system can get rid of it.

Seed in Hibernation

The herpes virus can live in the body undetected for years. This is like the seeds of certain trees which fall from the tree and bury themselves in the dirt for many years, waiting to sprout when the conditions are right. When your initial cold sore settles, the virus never actually goes away, it just hibernates like the seed, waiting for the right conditions. This can be when you have another infection or even if you are just feeling stressed.

Post-menopausal Hair Loss

Water-Scarce Garden

Like grass needs water to grow, your hair needs oestrogen. However, after menopause, you produce much less oestrogen. Just like a garden with a lack of water will lose a lot of grass, you lack oestrogen so you can lose a noticeable amount of hair.

Seborrheic Keratosis

Mud Stuck on Car

A seborrheic keratosis looks like a bit of mud stuck on your car. It might not look pleasant but it is harmless. We can choose to leave them stuck there or remove them for cosmetic purposes.

Skin

Rubber Band

Skin is like a rubber band. It becomes less elastic with age, and when exposed to heat it can deteriorate and crack.

Skin Cancer

Iceberg

Skin cancers can be like an iceberg – we can only see what is on the skin, but there is more below the surface. Some skin cancers are more likely to extend deeper below the surface than other cancers. This is why we can't just remove the cancer from the surface, we need to perform surgery and make sure we've removed all parts of the cancer, including the ones hiding deep in the skin. Other times, a piece of the iceberg can break off and float somewhere else. Similarly, cancer cells can spread from the main site to other parts of your skin and start to grow there.

Weed

Skin cancer is like a weed. It's easy to pull it off at the top, but it's essential to remove all the roots to make sure it won't just grow back again.

Skin Care

Working Out

To maintain healthy skin you need to consistently take care of it. It's like working out – you can't just lift weights one day, or only cleanse your skin one day, and expect to see any changes. You need to maintain it for a long period of time.

Symptomatic Treatment

Cooling Down an Overheated Car

Topical or symptomatic treatment of a condition is like pouring cold water over the hood of an overheated car. It may make the car feel colder, but it doesn't actually help the engine. For that, you need to go deeper and actually fix the problem.

Giving a Hungry Baby a Dummy

Topical or symptomatic treatment of a condition is like giving a hungry baby a dummy. It might placate them for a while, but eventually you will need to address the real issue.

Tinea Pedis (Athlete's Foot)

Moss Growing on Trees

Athlete's foot is like moss growing on trees, except it is on your skin. It is not enough to remove the moss from the surface of the tree, you need to continue treatment so you can kill the deeper roots and stop it growing again.

Vitiligo

Bleached Tee-Shirt

Vitiligo is like bleaching a coloured shirt, which causes it to lose its vibrant, bright or even dark colour, except instead of a shirt the colour is instead lost from your skin. This lost colour presents as areas of lighter coloured skin, just like a tee shirt that was only bleached in some parts.

Wound Care

Growing Plant

Caring for a wound is like caring for a plant. If you let the plant dry out or let the weeds flourish, it will not grow well. Similarly, we can't let the wound dry out or get too wet, and we need to remove any debris that might develop, such as pus.

Ear, Nose and Throat

Muhammad Azaan Khan, Gizem Ashraf,
Hamza Ashraf, Saad Ashraf,
Yusuf Hassan, Alisha Rawal,
Imaan Ashraf, Qazi Sarem Shahab,
and Zehra Hasimoglu

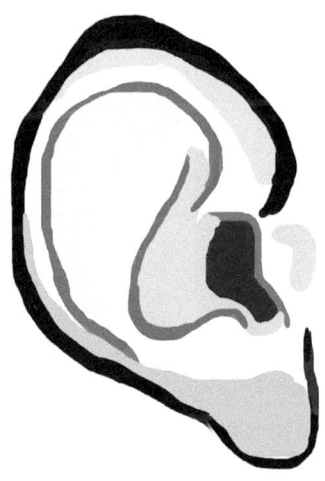

M. A. Khan (✉) · Q. S. Shahab
University of New South Wales, Sydney, NSW, Australia

G. Ashraf
Monash Health, Monash University, Melbourne, VIC, Australia

© The Author(s), under exclusive license to Springer Nature
Switzerland AG 2022
M. A. Khan et al. (eds.), *Medical Analogies for Clinician-Patient
Communication*, https://doi.org/10.1007/978-3-030-87293-9_3

H. Ashraf
Austin Health, Monash University, Melbourne, VIC, Australia

S. Ashraf · A. Rawal
Monash University, Clayton, VIC, Australia

Y. Hassan
The University of Melbourne, Melbourne, VIC, Australia

I. Ashraf
James Cook University, Douglas, QLD, Australia

Z. Hasimoglu
Latrobe University, Melbourne, VIC, Australia

Contents

Cholesteatoma

Blocked Drain

In cholesteatoma, there is an accumulation of skin cells within the middle ear. This accumulation of skin cells stops the ear from draining its gunk (discharge), which negatively affects the transmission of sound through the ear. This is just like how a blocked sink drain doesn't let things through. Additionally, like a blocked drain, there can be a foul smell and discharge coming from the ear.

Earwax Removal

Conveyor Belt

Your ear canal is like a conveyor belt. As wax builds up, the conveyor belt will push it out of the ear. This process might feel slow but if you use a cotton bud, you will push all the wax back up the belt and clog it up.

You can try gently washing out the ear canal in the shower, like a hose washing down the conveyor belt full of wax.

Otitis Media

Drum Full of Water

Your ear is like a drum. Usually hitting these drums makes a nice full sound. However, with otitis media, your ear is infected and full of bacteria and pus. This is like a drum being full of water. When you hit it, it doesn't vibrate well, which is why you cannot hear very well. Your eardrums can drain by themselves. This process can take a while, but if it doesn't correct itself we can try a few different things.

Sometimes, we need to shake the drum to help (Valsalva). At other times, we need to actually poke a hole in the drum to drain it. If this keeps happening and we do nothing, then the drum and everything inside will become rusty and no longer work. Similarly, your ear and hearing will become permanently damaged unless we treat it.

Sinus Surgery

Caves

The sinuses can be thought of as an intricate network of caves that have rivers flowing through them. The rivers are the natural secretions and mucus that your sinuses make, and if they do not flow out properly they are at risk of becoming infected. In sinus surgeries, we try to open up all the caves to make sure the rivers can flow out strongly and keep your sinuses clear.

Tonsillitis

Soldiers Overcrowding a Base

You have lymph nodes throughout your body. These are the bases or barracks for your white blood cells, which are the soldiers fighting against infection. When you have a throat infection, the lymph nodes in the throat, called the tonsils, go into alert mode and swell up with white blood cells. This is like how an army base would become very noisy and buzzing with soldiers running everywhere when there is an attack.

Endocrinology

4

Muhammad Azaan Khan, Gizem Ashraf,
Hamza Ashraf, Saad Ashraf,
Yusuf Hassan, Alisha Rawal,
Imaan Ashraf, Qazi Sarem Shahab,
and Zehra Hasimoglu

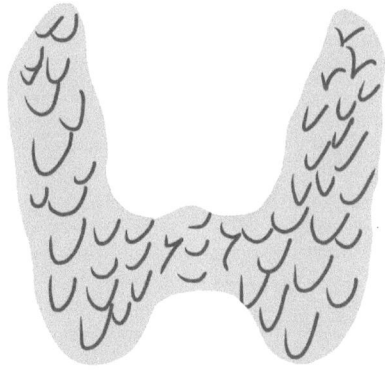

M. A. Khan (✉) · Q. S. Shahab
University of New South Wales, Sydney, NSW, Australia

G. Ashraf
Monash Health, Monash University, Melbourne, VIC, Australia

H. Ashraf
Austin Health, Monash University, Melbourne, VIC, Australia

© The Author(s), under exclusive license to Springer Nature
Switzerland AG 2022
M. A. Khan et al. (eds.), *Medical Analogies for Clinician-Patient
Communication*, https://doi.org/10.1007/978-3-030-87293-9_4

25

S. Ashraf · A. Rawal
Monash University, Clayton, VIC, Australia

Y. Hassan
The University of Melbourne, Melbourne, VIC, Australia

I. Ashraf
James Cook University, Douglas, QLD, Australia

Z. Hasimoglu
Latrobe University, Melbourne, VIC, Australia

Contents

Cushing's Syndrome – Thinning of Body Parts

Termites in a Wooden House

The impact of excess cortisol on your body is like letting termites loose in a wooden house. Like the wooden structures would be more hollow and bendable, patients experience thinning of skin, bones and muscles.

Bad Cement in the City

Your body has a type of tissue which holds everything together and functions as a strengthening anchor. This type of tissue is known as connective tissue, and it exists all over your body, particularly in your skin and bones. These cells are like the cement used to build a city, making the skyscrapers, pavements and pipes.

When you have Cushing syndrome, it is like the cement is going bad and losing its strength and quality. Slowly the city starts to fall apart, with the skyscrapers cracking, the pavement having holes and breaking up easily, and the water pipes bursting.

In your body, this means that the bones become less dense and crack more easily, like the skyscrapers; your skin becomes thin so healing is more difficult, like the crumbling pavement; and the extra water in your face and hypertension are from the water pipes being weak in places.

Steroid Weaning and Cessation

Sudden Stop While Driving

Imagine you are driving at a fast speed. If you wanted to stop, you would slowly apply the brakes and gradually come to a halt. That's what we are aiming to do when we stop using corticosteroids. If you were to go off the medication without slowly reducing the dose or frequency, it's analogous to slamming the brakes while you are going extremely fast. You've stopped the car, but that comes with significant damage to you and the car.

Dictator

Steroids are like a strong ruler who becomes a dictator. When there are problems in a country, sometimes a strong ruler is chosen because it is believed they will solve issues, just as we use a strong drug, steroids, to solve a problem in your body. If a dictator is allowed to enjoy power in the long run, they begin to misuse power, which wreaks havoc in the country. Similarly, long-term side effects of steroids can be quite damaging for the body. Another comparison that can be made between these two is the slow reduction of doses of steroids. Just as dictators don't give up their power immediately, suddenly ceasing the steroids doesn't work well for the body either. We need to slowly undermine the dictator's power, which is like gradually lowering the steroids dose, and eventually the steroid doses are small enough that we can just stop them.

Diabetes

Sugar Factory

Diabetes is a condition in which your body cannot control sugar. Normally, a hormone called insulin maintains strict control of your sugar levels. Insulin is like a sugar factory – it controls how much sugar is released into the blood. Higher levels of insulin allow the body's cells to take up sugar (glucose), which reduces the blood sugar levels. In diabetes, there is a problem with this sugar factory.

Type 1 diabetes is when the sugar factory (insulin) doesn't exist (no insulin) or works very poorly (little insulin production).

Type 2 diabetes is when the factory used to work well, but due to overuse it no longer functions properly. Sometimes it (insulin) works really fast (the cells take up glucose which reduces blood sugar levels) and sometimes really slow (the cells can't take up glucose which increases blood sugar levels).

Diabetes – Role of Insulin

Key to Open Building

Just like a building manager has a key which lets the workers in so they can start working on a building, the pancreas has a key (insulin) to let the sugar into the cells so they can work.

Diabetes – HbA1c

Donuts

HbA1c helps us measure your blood sugar levels. We all have red blood cells in our body. There are billions of them, and they look like donuts. In diabetic patients the amount of sugar on the donuts (red blood cells) is a lot more than usual. The more sugar there is, the worse the problem is.

Diabetes – Complications

Rodents

In diabetes, especially uncontrolled diabetes, there is a high level of sugar in the bloodstream. Imagine the nerves and blood vessels around your body as wiring and tubes. In complicated diabetes, the sugar deposits in these wires and tubes, thus attracting rodents to destroy and gnaw away at them. This is similar to your body's inflammatory response to the sugar deposits in the nerves and vessels causing irreversible damage.

Endocrine System

Spiderweb

The endocrine system is like a spiderweb. You cannot touch a single strand without affecting the rest of it.

Hormones

Car key

Hormones work by binding to receptors located throughout the body. Hormones are like car keys and receptors are like the ignition. Just as a key fits into the ignition, turns and starts the car's engines, hormones bind to receptors to activate them and start chemical reactions in the body. Just as cars only work with the right key, hormones can only bind to certain receptors. Hormones can either partially or fully activate a receptor. Partial activation is like using a car key to only turn on accessories like powering the windows or the radio. Full activation is like turning a key to start the engine. Just like a car can only act based on how far the key is turned, the body will act differently based on how the hormones are binding to receptors.

Hyperthyroidism and Hypothyroidism

Orchestra Conductor

The thyroid is like an orchestra conductor and the body is the orchestra.

Hypothyroidism is like a slow, sleepy conductor. Therefore, in hypothyroidism you feel tired, weak, depressed and slow in your movements and thoughts. Your body might also start gaining weight, become constipated and have muscle aches.

Hyperthyroidism is like a fast, overactive conductor. Therefore, in hyperthyroidism you feel anxious, irritable, hyperactive and tired. You might also feel sensitive to heat, have diarrhoea and muscle aches.

Steam Train

Your thyroid gland is like a steam train. If it consumes too much coal, it will go too fast – this is similar to how your body works too fast in hyperthyroidism. If it doesn't receive enough coal, then it won't go fast enough – this is similar to how your body is too slow in hypothyroidism.

Hypothyroidism

Spark Plug

The thyroid hormone is like the spark plug of the body. It is the spark which ignites the fuel to produce energy and allow the body to function. If the spark isn't there, it will be harder to ignite the fuel and therefore the body will be much slower – this is called hypothyroidism.

Metabolic Syndrome

Gang of Criminals

Think of the metabolic syndrome like a gang of criminals. For example, one of those criminals is your blood pressure, and another one is your blood sugar. Now each criminal itself can cause problems, like robbing a convenience store. But when the gang is together, they can cause more trouble, like robbing a bank. Each of them is individually a risk, but when they are together they make each other worse – the risk doesn't add up, it gets multiplied.

Similarly, hypertension is a risk factor for heart disease and diabetes is also a risk factor for heart disease, but when you have both, it makes it much more likely that you may develop heart disease. To fix the problem, we can't just catch one of the criminals, we need to catch all of the criminals to stop them from committing crime.

Osteoblast and Osteoclast Function

Tetris

Your osteoblasts produce bone, and your osteoclasts break down bone. It's like playing a game of Tetris. You add more blocks from the top, and the lines are destroyed at the bottom. You need to be adding blocks from the top but also losing blocks from the bottom otherwise you cannot win. Similarly, there needs to be a balance between bone production and bone destruction. Any imbalance can lead to weaker bones.

Osteoporosis

Termites

Osteoporosis for your body is like having a house with termites. It's a silent disease. You are not aware you have the termites until your house starts breaking apart. Similarly, it's often after a fracture that we diagnose the condition.

There are many management options, beginning with diet and exercise changes. We can also use certain medications, such as those which can slow the termites (slow breakdown of the bone) or those which can make the walls of the house strong (strength the bones).

Paraneoplastic Syndromes

Special Remote

Paraneoplastic syndromes are like special remotes which can control various features in your home. Although the main reason you might have bought your remote was to control the TV, you can also install extra features like switching your lights or heating on. Most cancers are like standard remotes that can only impact the TV or one part of your body, but some cancers impact additional things such as your hormones. We call these paraneoplastic syndromes.

Pituitary Tumour

Specialised Factory

Think of your pituitary gland like a factory with many specialised departments that produce different hormones. Now imagine a pituitary tumour is like one department that randomly starts to expand. It takes over the adjacent department and the next. It's unstoppable. As it expands, it shuts down the function of all those departments it takes over, causing a deficiency in some hormones and a dangerous excess of one hormone. Depending on which department is taking over, the effects of the pituitary tumour changes.

Additionally, the factory has several structures around it. In this case, we are concerned about the structures around the pituitary gland, in particular, the nerves around the gland that function as specialised electrical wires responsible for your eyesight. If the factory continues to expand due to the over-enthusiastic department, the electrical wires may be compressed and thus cause visual defects. This is how a pituitary adenoma can cause you to see as if you're wearing horse blinders.

Pituitary and Thyroid Gland Interaction

Thermostat and Air-Conditioner

Your thyroid is like an air-conditioner. It can make things hotter or colder. However, the air-conditioner is controlled by the thermostat, which senses the temperature of the environment and makes changes to the air-conditioner. Similarly, the pituitary gland senses changes in the body and makes adjustments to the level of hormones secreted by the thyroid gland.

Total thyroidectomy and Thyroxine Replacement

Shutting Down the Factory

Imagine your thyroid as a factory. If the amount of the hormones that the thyroid is producing in your body is too high, we need to shut down part of the factory. We do this by removing part or all of the thyroid.

Once your thyroid is removed and the factory is no longer working, we need to import the product from an external source because your body still needs thyroid hormone, which we can give as a medication.

Thyroid: Radioactive Iodine Therapy

Trojan Horse

Most of the iodine that enters the body is taken up by the thyroid cells. The thyroid cancer cells are especially overactive and take up lots of iodine. Therefore, we can target them by utilsing radioactive iodine, which when administered acts like a trojan horse and is taken in by the cancer cells and destroys them from inside. This helps mop any cancer cells that might have been left behind or have spread.

Gastroenterology

5

Muhammad Azaan Khan, Gizem Ashraf,
Hamza Ashraf, Saad Ashraf,
Yusuf Hassan, Alisha Rawal,
Imaan Ashraf, Qazi Sarem Shahab,
and Zehra Hasimoglu

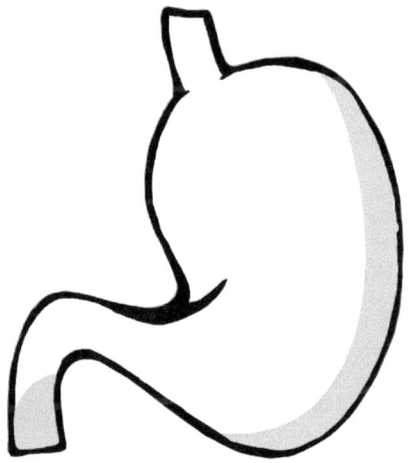

M. A. Khan (✉) · Q. S. Shahab
University of New South Wales, Sydney, NSW, Australia

G. Ashraf
Monash Health, Monash University, Melbourne, VIC, Australia

© The Author(s), under exclusive license to Springer Nature
Switzerland AG 2022
M. A. Khan et al. (eds.), *Medical Analogies for Clinician-Patient
Communication*, https://doi.org/10.1007/978-3-030-87293-9_5

H. Ashraf
Austin Health, Monash University, Melbourne, VIC, Australia

S. Ashraf · A. Rawal
Monash University, Clayton, VIC, Australia

Y. Hassan
The University of Melbourne, Melbourne, VIC, Australia

I. Ashraf
James Cook University, Douglas, QLD, Australia

Z. Hasimoglu
Latrobe University, Melbourne, VIC, Australia

Contents

Chronic Liver Disease and Cirrhosis

Old Donkey

Your liver is like a plodding donkey that is old and sick and carries on without complaining, until it is too late. On the other hand, your heart or your lungs, which can be compared to a baby that cries every time it is hungry or tired or sick, shows its symptoms, such as chest pain or shortness of breath.

Coeliac Disease

Smoking Cigarettes

Eating gluten might cause you to have symptoms like abdominal pain and diarrhoea which may not appear serious but in the long term it also increases your risk of cancer. Just like we know that smoking cigarettes causes lung cancer, eating gluten increases the risk of cancer for patients with coeliac disease. Some people might find smoking to be enjoyable just as you might enjoy eating gluten, but each time you eat gluten you are increasing your risk.

Gastroenteritis

Security Measures – Emergency Escape Button and Sweating Out Bugs

Your gut is a tightly regulated system that has its own security system patrolling it constantly to ensure no dangerous substances or bacteria enter and destroy the system. One of the safety mechanisms of the security system is the emergency escape button that ejects all contents of the gut from both ends: resulting in either vomiting or diarrhoea. Another security measure against bacteria is to raise the temperature of the body, which induces a fever so that the bacteria can't survive.

Gastro-Oesophageal Reflux Disease (GORD) – Symptomatic Management

Paracetamol for Headache

If someone has a headache occasionally, they only take paracetamol when they get the headache, instead of all the time. Similarly, you do not need to take proton pump inhibitor (PPI) all the time, only when you have symptoms of GORD. If you have symptoms every day, then your doctor might tell you to take PPI every day.

Hepatitis Dormancy

Underground Coup

Think of the hepatitis virus like a criminal network infiltrating a government. They start off underground and slowly build their numbers. At this stage they cause a little bit of trouble, but not too much damage. The virus does the same thing, slowly replicating and building up its numbers.

Once they get enough members, the criminal network launches an all-out attack on the government – this is what we call acute hepatitis, or inflammation of the liver. Your body or the government responds and fights the criminal network. Eventually it gets it under control. Then, either the criminal network can build its numbers again and launch another attack, or the government can completely get rid of every member of the network so it can't cause any problems. Similarly, the hepatitis virus can remain dormant and potentially cause other acute attacks later on in life.

Hepatitis – Phases

Park Ranger Trying to Capture a Wild Bear

The different stages of infection can be compared to a park ranger trying to capture a wild bear.

The first stage is the silent stage, also known as the immune tolerant stage, because the immune system is not responding to the virus/bear. In this stage, the bear is just hibernating and not actively doing anything and therefore the park ranger is not aware of it.

The second stage is the damage phase, also known as the immune clearance stage, where your immune system starts to clear the virus and fights back, causing damage. It's as if the sleeping bear has come out of hibernation and the park ranger is fighting it.

The third stage is the control stage, also known as the immune control stage. This is where the park ranger has captured the bear and put it in a cage. The bear is still there but has been controlled. Similarly, the virus is still in the body but has been controlled by the immune system.

A fourth stage that can occur is the escape stage, also known as the immune escape phase. This happens when the bear escapes the cage and causes damage again, just like the virus can multiply again and cause damage to the liver.

The fifth and final stage is the clear stage, where the body has been cleared of the virus completely. This is similar to the park ranger putting the bear down so it can't return to cause damage. Of course, another bear can come along, which happens if you get re-infected, and then the stages start again.

Inflammatory Bowel Disease (IBD)

Rugged Road

Imagine very severe rainfall on a badly constructed road. It's going to be riddled with potholes. Travelling through the road will be bumpy, annoying to drive on, may damage the car, and driving on this poorly road may even break the road more. Your intestines have become like this road because of inflammation. Food 'driving' through this tract causes a lot of bumps and is irritating, which is why it hurts after meals, and there are periods of diarrhoea and constipation.

Irritable Bowel Syndrome (IBS) – Pathophysiology

Toothpaste Tube

Your bowel is similar to a long tube of toothpaste. In a normally functioning bowel, you squeeze toothpaste from one end to the other end, and it comes out in a nice regular way. In IBS, the toothpaste is squeezed from multiple points at the same time as opposed to from one end to the other, which means the stool doesn't come out nicely, which causes pressure to build up and therefore pain.

Irritable Bowel Syndrome (IBS) – Management

Leg Cramps

Leg cramps are very real and very painful, but they don't occur because there is something seriously wrong with your legs, it is because your muscles aren't behaving properly. The same goes for your irritable bowels – it is definitely a real and painful condition, but it isn't because of a serious underlying problem; rather, the bowels are misbehaving, what also explains why the tests are normal but you are still experiencing the pain.

This means we don't have anything to fix or cure; however, we need to manage bowels better overall. We do not perform interventions on muscles for leg cramps, such as surgery, but we can use conservative lifestyle measures such as stretching, exercise, etc. Similarly, there is no intervention in IBS – we just need to adopt conservative lifestyle measures.

Irritable Bowel Syndrome (IBS) – Normal Investigation Results

Headache

IBS is like a headache. If you examined every part of the body in someone with a headache they would probably look normal, but they still have the very real pain. Sometimes you have pain and it doesn't cause a physical or observable change in your body.

Jaundice

Toilet and Water Inside the Bowl

Imagine your liver as a toilet that removes waste products. Usually toilet water is clear; however, sometimes it can become discoloured with waste products. In your body, we assess the colour of this 'toilet water' or liver function through the clarity of your eyes and skin. However, the toilet water can become discoloured in a number of ways.

Firstly, if there is a plumbing blockage downstream from the toilet, no matter how many times you flush, the toilet water will always be discoloured. This is similar to when you have gallstones causing a blockage downstream from your liver.

Secondly, if your toilet is broken and can't flush the waste well enough, the toilet water will also become discoloured. This is what happens when your liver is attacked by a virus or chronically damaged and causes build-up of the waste products.

Lastly, if there is more waste than the toilet can flush out, the toilet water will remain discoloured, similar to when the liver is overwhelmed with waste products and can't clear them fast enough, resulting in eye and skin yellowing.

Liver Disease – Alcoholic

Sponge

The liver is like the body's sponge. When you clean a very dirty or oily dish, the sponge also becomes grimy, and over time it eventually no longer works very well. This is similar to what happens when you consume a lot of alcohol or fatty foods. The liver does its job at the start; however, it becomes dirty and soiled from the cleaning. Eventually, it becomes so damaged that it has wrinkled up and is no longer functional, like an old sponge, which we call liver disease.

Liver Failure

Massive Factory

Your liver is like a massive factory which is responsible for a whole country. This factory makes many important things, like proteins and bile. It also has a large processing centre, which looks at many of the things in your body and decides what to do with them. In liver failure, this factory stops manufacturing all of its products and stops processing what's in your body. If the factory doesn't return to normal, the whole body can be affected.

Opportunistic Infections

Troublesome Teenagers Causing Major Problems

Every neighbourhood has some troublesome teenagers that loiter around, but with a few police officers present, they never cause serious trouble. Now imagine if all the police officers were recruited to a major fight elsewhere in the city or were wiped out completely for other reasons. The troublesome teenagers will now take over the neighbourhood and cause serious damage without any authorities to intervene. Similarly, your gut has some resident bugs that usually cause no harm; but if your immunity is down, these bugs can cause some serious problems.

Peptic Ulcer Disease

Tug of War

Think of your stomach as being in a constant tug of war with a good and bad side. Imagine the bad side winning as an ulcer forming – slowly the bad side starts pulling harder and harder so the ulcer gets bigger and worse. At the end, they make one last strong pull and the good side falls over. This is the ulcer 'winning' and eroding through the entire stomach wall.

With a *Helicobacter pylori* infection, it's like adding Arnold Schwarzenegger to the bad side's team, making them much more likely to win.

When you take a lot of NSAIDs, it's like pouring water underneath the good side's team, now it's really hard for them to win and they'll slip and lose.

To make it easier for the good guys to win, we can give medication which gets rid of some of the bad guys. However, if you stop taking the medication, the bad guys that we got rid of will come back and the bad side will win again.

Stool Consistency – Normal Population Variation

Variations in Bananas

Bowel motions can have different consistencies and still be normal, just like bananas can have different consistencies and still be normal. Some people like very green, hard and unripe, others like yellow and soft, and some prefer brown and overripe and mushy. It all depends on what you personally prefer, as long as it is within the range of normal. Abnormal is like eating a banana that is half-grown, or when it has turned black and mouldy.

General Practice

6

Muhammad Azaan Khan, Gizem Ashraf,
Hamza Ashraf, Saad Ashraf,
Yusuf Hassan, Alisha Rawal,
Imaan Ashraf, Qazi Sarem Shahab,
and Zehra Hasimoglu

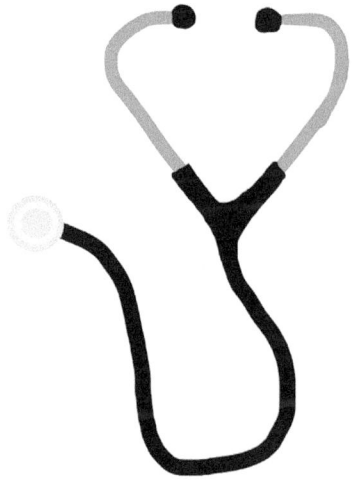

M. A. Khan (✉) · Q. S. Shahab
University of New South Wales, Sydney, NSW, Australia

G. Ashraf
Monash Health, Monash University, Melbourne, VIC, Australia

© The Author(s), under exclusive license to Springer Nature
Switzerland AG 2022
M. A. Khan et al. (eds.), *Medical Analogies for Clinician-Patient
Communication*, https://doi.org/10.1007/978-3-030-87293-9_6

H. Ashraf
Austin Health, Monash University, Melbourne, VIC, Australia

S. Ashraf · A. Rawal
Monash University, Clayton, VIC, Australia

Y. Hassan
The University of Melbourne, Melbourne, VIC, Australia

I. Ashraf
James Cook University, Douglas, QLD, Australia

Z. Hasimoglu
Latrobe University, Melbourne, VIC, Australia

Contents

Antibiotics for Viral Infections

Cockroach Spray Versus Cockroach Spray

Imagine you have a possum living in the roof of your house so you call the pest removal service. They tell you that they don't have the right thing to get rid of the possum and it will probably just leave on its own in a week or so. It wouldn't then make sense to ask them for cockroach spray to spray in the roof to get rid of the possum.

Asking for antibiotics for a viral infection is like asking for cockroach spray to get rid of a possum. It won't do anything to the possum, but instead you will need to deal with the extra unnecessary chemicals, and you will still need to wait for the possum to leave on its own anyway.

Discharge Planning (for Non-surgical Cases)

Postoperative Hospital Stay

After a patient has surgery, the treating team doesn't send them home immediately. The patient is given time in hospital to allow their wound to start healing. Although you have not had surgery, we have adjusted your medications and also need to give your body time to adjust and stabilise before we send you home.

Education and Awareness

Flashlight in the Dark

Understanding your illness may help you manage it better. For example, in the dark it's difficult to differentiate between a rope and a snake but a flashlight would help you. Adequate knowledge about an illness can act as a flashlight in helping differentiate your symptoms from normal experiences. We need to shine a light to better understand what is going on.

Inconsistent Medication Use

Unwatered Plant

When you stop watering a plant, the plant doesn't die immediately. However, once it dies you need to start from the start with a new seed. Similarly, if you don't take your medications regularly, you can lose the health benefits of the medication and need to start from scratch.

Boiling Water

For water to boil, we need to keep the stove on until it starts bubbling. However, if we keep turning the stove on and off it's never going to become hot enough to boil. Your medication is like the stove; just like the stove needs to remain on continuously, you need to keep taking medications regularly otherwise you will never see results.

Latent Viruses

Seeds

Some seeds stay hidden in the ground for many years until the conditions are right for them to sprout. Similarly, some viruses can stay hidden in your body and only become a problem if the conditions are right.

Long-Term Medications

Eyeglasses

Once patients feel like they have recovered, they sometimes believe they no longer need to continue their medication. However, the medication will stop working if you stop taking it. For example, people who wear glasses are able to see clearly when their glasses are on but if they throw their glasses away, they will no longer be able to see clearly. Similarly, you feel well because you are taking your medication regularly. If you stop the medication, you will not be as well and the medication can lose its effect completely, as if you never took it in the first place.

Management of Healthcare Workers

Surgeon Self-Operating

No matter how experienced a surgeon is, they can't operate on themselves. Similarly, although you might be aware of your symptoms and knowledgeable about the treatment, you still need to let others help you.

Medications When Asymptomatic

Locking the Door

Every day when you leave your home you lock the door. You don't do this because there are thieves waiting; you do it to avoid the risk of being robbed. Similarly, your medications keep you safe and minimise the risk of you becoming unwell, even if you feel perfectly fine right now.

Non-compliance

Not Servicing Your Car

Just because you don't service your car once and it doesn't cause trouble, it doesn't mean it will continue to function properly. Similarly, if you're lucky once or twice to not experience symptoms of relapse when non-compliant with your medications, this does not mean that this will always be the case. The risk of relapse does not decrease, and that is why it is important to comply with your treatment plan.

Not Completing the Full Course of Antibiotics

Special Weapon

When you're sick, your body is fighting against whatever is making it sick. You will use different weapons depending on the battle.

On day one of the battle you will wipe out most of the bad guys, but some will still be left behind. On day two, you'll wipe out some more and only a few of the bad guys are left behind. You might be feeling better so you don't keep fighting.

But the ones you left behind are the most resistant of them all and if you leave them alone, they are able to build up their own army. The next time you fight the battle, the bad guys are stronger and have worked out a way to survive against your weapon. So your weapon is no longer effective.

This is what happens when we inappropriately use antibiotics and do not complete the required course. The bugs we leave behind are resistant to our antibiotics and they reproduce and become a superbug version of the original, less harmful bug.

Firefighters

Antibiotics are like firefighters. If your house was burning the fire-fighters wouldn't just stop when the large flames and smoke has settled, they would also want to douse the embers as well, otherwise the fire will restart and may be harder to control. Similarly your symptoms may have settled but there are still remnants of the bugs, and if we don't douse them out with antibiotics they will overrun your body again!

Not Seeing Improvement

Uphill Journey

The path to a destination at the top of the hill is often not straight, easy or short. At times you may feel you are not making any progress but with every step you are getting closer to your destination. Similarly, your treatment and ongoing efforts are bringing us closer to our goal of a healthier you.

Boiling Water

Not seeing any improvement despite all of your treatment is like trying to boil water. Although we can't see it, the water is getting hotter and hotter and eventually, we will see when it boils. Your treatment is helping in the same way, and eventually it too will show results.

Patient-Centred Care

Coach and Star-Player

Managing a condition is not something we do to the patient – it's something we do with the patient. The doctor is the coach, and the patient is the star-player. The doctor and patient work together to decide the game plan. Throughout the game, if the player feels like the chosen plan or treatment is not working, they will let the coach know to revise the strategy. A coach would never send their star-player into a tough game without knowing or understanding the game plan. Similarly, the doctor must maintain communication with the patient about the treatment plan to ensure the best possible outcome.

Preventative Care – Reducing Severity

Seatbelt

We take these steps for preventative management. When you are in a car you wear a seat belt. You know this won't prevent an accident from happening but if one does happen, your injuries will be much less severe. Similarly, we can institute preventative management to decrease the severity of the outcome if something goes wrong.

Slow-Acting Medications

Fruit Growth

Waiting for medical treatment to act is like waiting for fruit to grow. A farmer plants his seeds and waits. It might take days before there is any growth and weeks before there is any fruit. Similarly, some medications take time to act in the body.

Unnecessary Imaging

Coffee and Sugar

If we took a photo of a cup of coffee it wouldn't tell us how much sugar is in the coffee. We can only know this by tasting the coffee. A scan may give us more information but at other times, no matter how many pictures we take, we won't get any more information – for that, we actually need to taste it, or in this case, biopsy it.

General Surgery

7

Hamza Ashraf, Muhammad Azaan Khan,
Gizem Ashraf, Saad Ashraf, Yusuf Hassan,
Alisha Rawal, Imaan Ashraf,
Qazi Sarem Shahab,
and Zehra Hasimoglu

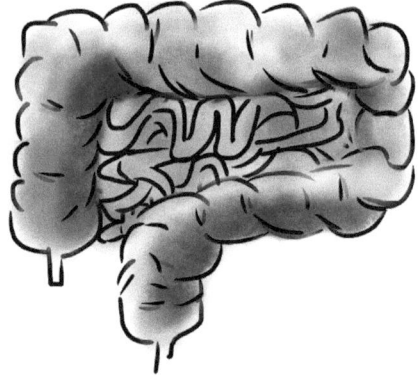

H. Ashraf
Austin Health, Monash University, Melbourne, VIC, Australia

M. A. Khan (✉) · Q. S. Shahab
University of New South Wales, Sydney, NSW, Australia

G. Ashraf
Monash Health, Monash University, Melbourne, VIC, Australia

© The Author(s), under exclusive license to Springer Nature
Switzerland AG 2022
M. A. Khan et al. (eds.), *Medical Analogies for Clinician-Patient
Communication*, https://doi.org/10.1007/978-3-030-87293-9_7

S. Ashraf · A. Rawal
Monash University, Clayton, VIC, Australia

Y. Hassan
The University of Melbourne, Melbourne, VIC, Australia

I. Ashraf
James Cook University, Douglas, QLD, Australia

Z. Hasimoglu
Latrobe University, Melbourne, VIC, Australia

Contents

Achalasia

Stuck Gate on the Road

Your oesophagus is the road carrying food from your mouth to your stomach. Right before the stomach, it has to get past the sphincter, which is a gate which opens only when food is passing through. In achalasia, this gate becomes stuck, so it's hard to open. This means the traffic, your food, can't go into the stomach and can build up in the oesophagus, which can cause issues.

Appendicitis

Janitor Closet at an Airport

Everyone at an airport goes from the main gate to the plane in an orderly fashion, from one end of the terminal to the other. This is like your stool moving from one end of your bowels to the other, and the plane taking off is when you defecate. Imagine if one person becomes lost on his way to the terminal and ends up in the janitor side-closet, and then gets stuck, thereby blocking it off.

This is when a small stone called a faecolith blocks off a side-exit in your bowel called the appendix.

Now the janitor can't get to his cleaning materials, which means slowly the rest of the airport will become dirty and more people will begin to get clogged up. This is similar to how the appendix gets inflamed and can spread that inflammation to the rest of the abdomen.

Biliary Colic

Tomato Sauce Bottle

Your gallbladder is similar to a tomato sauce bottle, which squeezes the sauce onto your food when it's time to eat to make it more palatable. Similarly, your gallbladder squeezes its juices into your intestine when it's time to eat to make your food more digestible.

However, if you have something blocking the exit of the tomato sauce bottle, for example if you twist the lid shut, then firstly the sauce won't get out, and secondly if you squeeze the bottle it will cause pressure to build up inside. Similarly, if you have gallstones blocking the exit, every time your gallbladder squeezes at food time the pressure will build up and will cause pain. This is called biliary colic.

Bowel Cancer Screening

Car Warning Lights

A screening test is much like a car warning light. A flashing warning light doesn't tell you what is wrong with the engine. In the same way that it is possible for multiple things to be wrong with a car engine, it is possible for multiple conditions to cause blood in the stool. This means that a positive screening test result does not mean you have bowel cancer. A closer look, like a diagnostic test, is needed to definitively diagnose or exclude bowel cancer. The warning light only indicates that something may be wrong. It is also possible for the screening test to return a false positive: to pick out someone without an issue at all. This would be like the car warning light flashing due to a problem with the sensor itself, despite the engine being fine.

Bowel Infarction

Heart Attack for the Bowel

Every organ needs a blood supply to survive. But when this supply line is blocked, the part of the organ beyond that blockage dies. This is classically seen in a heart attack, where the blood supply to the heart is blocked. However, less commonly, this can happen to one's bowel, resulting in dead bowel if the supply line isn't restored quickly enough.

Cholecystectomy – Fat Metabolism

Washing Oily Dishes Without Soap

Your gallbladder stores bile, which is like detergent. Trying to digest fatty food without your gallbladder is like trying to wash greasy dishes without any detergent – it's quite difficult. That's why you might have some trouble digesting fatty foods.

Colorectal Cancer

Journey on a Long Road

Think of the development of colorectal cancer as a long road. The first part of the journey is when there are abnormal changes in the cells of your colon. The end destination is colorectal cancer. There are many stops along the way and you can stop your journey at any of those points. When you have tests done, we find out how far along the road you have come and if you're nearing the final destination that is colorectal cancer.

When approaching the final destination, cars begin to break down and release smoke as a warning sign of bad things to come. Similarly, your bowel can bleed in small amounts as a warning sign it's heading for a cancerous destination. When you have a treatment, such as surgery, you turn back around on the road towards safety or even return right to the beginning.

Constipation – Cancerous

Blocked Traffic

Constipation is like a traffic jam. In some circumstances, the road can be blocked due to an obstruction. Sometimes this can happen suddenly, like a tree falling onto the road, blocking traffic. Or the tree can start out as a seedling making cracks in the road. This seedling grows and grows, causing an increasing number of traffic jams as it branches across the road. After some time you end up with a massive tree in the middle of the road blocking all traffic. This is like a bowel cancer insidiously growing over time and causing worsening constipation and eventually a bowel obstruction.

Constipation – Drug-Induced

Roadworks

Medications are used to fix things in the body, just like roadworks fix road problems. However, an unwanted consequence of roadworks is slowing down traffic. Similarly, some medications slow down your bowel motions whilst they do their repairs.

Constipation – Slow Transit

Traffic Jam

Constipation is like a traffic jam. There may be nothing wrong with the road or with the cars, but the speed limit is just too low, which causes the hold-up.

Diverticular Disease

Potholes

Think of your digestive tract as a long road. If the road is smooth, then food can travel through without any trouble. However, roads can have potholes, which slow down transit and can even cause accidents. In your digestive tract, these potholes are diverticula, and they can cause blockages, inflammation and pain as food and stool passes through and get stuck there.

Fibre and Bulk Laxatives

Sponge

Fibre and bulk laxatives are like a sponge. It absorbs water from its surroundings and draws it into the bowel to make the stool soft. This is why you need to drink water with your fibre – if you have fibre without water, then the sponge won't have any water to absorb so it won't do its job and consequently the stool won't be soft.

Fissure

Paper Cut

An anal fissure is like a small papercut in your anus. Sometimes they can hurt even when resting, but most of the time a papercut hurts most when it comes into contact with something painful, like soap when you wash your hands. Similarly, anal fissures will hurt most when they come into contact with hard constipated stool as you try to pass stool, causing intense pain. To let a papercut heal you need to let it rest, which means to stop irritating it with soap. Similarly, you need to let the fissure heal, which we do by stopping it from coming into contact with hard constipated stool. This means you need to keep your stool soft.

Fistula

Unwanted Connection Between Two Separate Train Tunnels

Your body is filled with many specialised train tunnels, stool and urine for example. Usually, these train tunnels do not connect with each other in order to keep things nicely specialised. However, for many different reasons, be it physical damage or congenital abnormalities, these tunnels can connect, causing the wrong substances to travel down the wrong tunnels.

Haemorrhoids

Varicose Veins

Just as varicose veins are those veins that don't work properly in your legs and fill up with blood and swell, haemorrhoids also occur when the veins in your anus don't work properly and fill up with blood and swell. When they are small neither of them hurt, but when varicose veins and haemorrhoids get bigger, then the pressure inside can cause pain.

Hernia

Inner Tube of Tyre

We can think of a hernia as the inner tube of a tyre bulging out through the surface of a damaged tyre. Similarly, when the abdominal wall weakens like the surface of the damaged tyre, the bowel can push through the weakening and make a bulge like the inner tube of the tyre.

To fix the problem, we need to firstly push the inner tube (the bowel) back in, and then repair the damage on the surface of the tyre, which is repairing the hole in the abdominal wall with some mesh.

Mallory–Weiss Tear

Oesophagus is a Rubber Band

Think of your oesophagus as a rubber band. When you stretch a rubber band aggressively, it gets weaker and might develop little tears. After binge drinking and vomiting a lot, especially if you do this often, you can develop little tears in your oesophagus, which we call Mallory–Weiss tears.

Pancreatic Cancer

Old Donkey

Your pancreas can lose 90% of its function before your body shows any symptoms. In this way, your pancreas is like a plodding donkey that carries on without complaining even when it gets old and sick until it is too late. This is why in many cases pancreatic cancer is detected late. On the other hand, your heart or your lungs, which can be compared to a child which cries whenever it is hungry or tired or sick, acutely complain and show their symptoms, such as chest pain or shortness of breath.

Pancreatitis

Factory on the Road

Imagine there is a road in your body: on one end of the road you have the pancreas and on the other end you have the gallbladder and liver. The pancreas is like a factory that produces important substances for your body and through the road, or biliary tree, is connected to the gallbladder and liver.

In pancreatitis, the factory is damaged. This can be caused by damage to the factory itself or a problem in another part of the road, like in the gallbladder. For example, gallstones block and damage the road leading to the pancreas causing issues with the pancreas itself.

If the factory was damaged or on fire, the contents of the factory spill outside. We know that your factory, your pancreas, has a problem because the levels of substances produced in the pancreas and other surrounding areas along the road (the pancreas, gallbladder, and the liver) are abnormal and leaking into the bloodstream.

Peritonitis

Electric Fence

The abdomen has linings which enclose and secure everything inside, similar to an electric fence. Normally it isn't on and touching it doesn't hurt. When we have infection, the fence turns on and it hurts to touch.

Post-Operative Ileus

Scared Turtle

Picture a scared turtle. The scared turtle is going to hang out in its shell, not moving, until it feels safe again. You can't bribe it back out. Your bowels act like this scared turtle, when they are threatened (for example after a surgery). The bowel stops moving its muscles and is just waiting for a time when it feels the threat has passed.

Haematology

8

Muhammad Azaan Khan, Gizem Ashraf,
Hamza Ashraf, Saad Ashraf,
Yusuf Hassan, Alisha Rawal,
Imaan Ashraf, Qazi Sarem Shahab,
and Zehra Hasimoglu

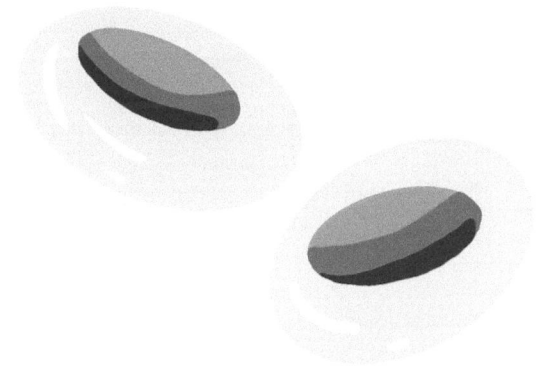

M. A. Khan (✉) · Q. S. Shahab
University of New South Wales, Sydney, NSW, Australia

G. Ashraf
Monash Health, Monash University, Melbourne, VIC, Australia

H. Ashraf
Austin Health, Monash University, Melbourne, VIC, Australia

S. Ashraf · A. Rawal
Monash University, Clayton, VIC, Australia

Y. Hassan
The University of Melbourne, Melbourne, VIC, Australia

I. Ashraf
James Cook University, Douglas, QLD, Australia

Z. Hasimoglu
Latrobe University, Melbourne, VIC, Australia

Contents

Anaemia

Trucks

You have red blood cells which carry oxygen and nutrients to your body so it can use them. They are like delivery trucks which take the groceries from the farm to the different supermarkets.

Imagine if the trucks were leaving the farm without being fully loaded. The supermarkets would be emptier and eventually people would complain and starve. This is what happens in anaemia. Your red blood cells are not fully packed with oxygen, so your body is not getting all the groceries it needs, causing it to become tired.

There can be a lot of reasons why red blood cells aren't full of oxygen. The trucks might not be full because they don't have enough fuel or enough crew members to load the trucks or because some trucks break down a lot. The trucks might not be full because something might be wrong at the farm; for example, a lack of fertiliser, meaning not enough groceries can be made. This is similar to missing an important nutrient in the body, for example, iron deficiency, which can cause anaemia.

Bleeding Disorders

Dam

If you have a strong dam made of rocks and cement, a small trauma to the dam might only let a little bit of water through. The dam represents your body's ability to form a clot with platelets and the water represents blood. In patients with bleeding disorders, trauma to the dam doesn't only let a little bit of water through but actually results in the dam bursting which means you bleed a lot.

Clotting Cascade

Dominos

The clotting cascade is like a line of dominos. If one domino is missing it impacts the entire line. Similarly, if your body is deficient in one clotting factor it will slow down the entire clotting process.

Coagulopathy

Beavers Making a Dam

When you've cut yourself on something and start bleeding, your body instantly tries to patch up the hole. This is like beavers building a dam whenever they see a stream of water. But when you have a bleeding disorder, it means that the patch your body is trying to make isn't strong enough. This is like if the beavers didn't have enough wood, or the wood was very weak and had a lot of holes in it. In your case, you don't have enough of a certain substance, which is like the beavers not having enough wood to patch the bleed quickly; hence, it takes longer to make a clot.

Leaking Boat

When you've cut yourself on something and start bleeding, your body instantly tries to patch up the hole. This is like a boat and you patch up leaks in the hull as they pop up. But when you have a bleeding disorder, it means that the patch your body is trying to make isn't strong enough. This is as if you didn't have all the materials right away or manpower to patch the hole in the boat. Therefore, it takes longer for the leak in the boat to be patched, just as it takes longer for you to stop bleeding.

Deep Vein Thrombosis (DVT) and Pulmonary Embolism (PE)

Rotten Milk

A DVT is when you have a clot in one of your deep leg veins. Your blood that has clotted is like milk that has thickened and curdled. Imagine trying to pour that milk. As you keep pouring, eventually the curds at the bottom will go to the mouth of the bottle and get stuck, so you can't pour any more. This can happen to your lungs – all the blood from your legs eventually goes to your lungs but suddenly the flow stops because you've got a big clot blocking it.

To keep allowing flow, we need to remove the curd – or in your case, the clot. We either do this by breaking it up using medication or manually removing it. Then, we need to find out why the milk is going bad and thickening to form curds, which means finding out why your blood is thickening easily and forming clots.

Iron, B12, Folate Deficiency

Delivery Van

Your body transports oxygen in the blood via red blood cells – think of these as delivery vans that drop oxygen off at cells. Just as a van is made from various materials, so too are red blood cells; in particular iron, B12 and folate. However, if you lacked the basic materials, such as steel, glass and plastic, you'll build fewer vans and thus you'd have less delivery ability. Similarly, if you don't have enough of these basic building blocks, your body won't make as many red blood cells, and decrease its oxygen transport capacity.

Leukaemia

The Flower Garden

Your bones contain bone marrow, which is constantly producing different cells for your bloodstream. These are the red blood cells for oxygen, white blood cells for protection against infection, and platelets for stopping bleeding. Think of bone marrow as the soil of a garden, and all of those different cells as the different seeds and roots for the grass, flowers and trees. Sometimes, there can be an invasion of the garden soil by weeds, resulting in the garden being filled with useless weeds rather than grass, flowers and trees. Similarly, leukaemia is a cancer, an overgrowth, of a bone marrow cell which reduces the production of the important blood cells.

Lymphadenopathy

Fire Station

Think of lymph nodes as a fire station. You don't notice them normally, but as soon as there is a threat, they go into action mode: alarms are blaring, people are running all over the site, and there is a lot of activity there. Your lymph nodes are now in their action mode, which is causing them to swell up, and are working hard to put out the infection.

Lymphoma

Malfunctioning Military Training Camps

There are several types of immune cells in the body which protect us against infection, each with a different role. This is similar to how there are different service jobs like the police, military, air force and navy. Two important cell types are B cells, which make antibodies – these are like soldiers with rifles – and T cells, which coordinate how the immune system responds and also kill infected cells directly – these are like high-ranking generals.

In lymphoma, there may be a malfunction in the production of one of these cells, usually the B cells. The boot camp for these cells or soldiers is usually very stressful and hard, so only qualified and healthy soldiers make it through. It also trains them and makes them stronger. Our body does the same thing to mature our B and T immune cells, but this training camp is in the lymph nodes. However, if the training camp malfunctions, then immature soldiers can make it through, as seen in lymphoma where many cancerous, immature, immune cells are produced and cause harm to the body instead of helping it.

School

Every child goes to school and learns skills which they can then use to get a job. Imagine if schools stopped teaching and only filled their hours with free time. None of the children would know anything for their exams, and would continually repeat their year. Your immune cells are like these children. They go to a place like school, which for them, are your lymph nodes, where they mature and learn their role in protecting you from infections. In lymphoma, it's as if the school stopped teaching – or in your case, the body has stopped teaching the immune cells how to do their job. So they just keep staying in the lymph nodes, like the children repeating their years of school. This is bad because eventually there are too many children failing and the schools can't take in anymore – so what do those kids do? They become hooligans and loiter where they shouldn't be. Your immune cells eventually do the same and spread throughout the body, like the brain, liver or kidney.

Infectious Diseases

9

Muhammad Azaan Khan, Gizem Ashraf,
Hamza Ashraf, Saad Ashraf,
Yusuf Hassan, Alisha Rawal,
Imaan Ashraf, Qazi Sarem Shahab,
and Zehra Hasimoglu

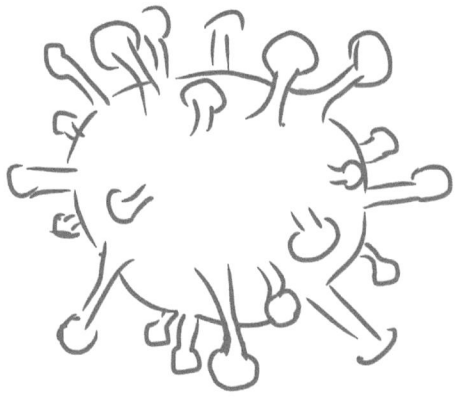

M. A. Khan (✉) · Q. S. Shahab
University of New South Wales, Sydney, NSW, Australia

G. Ashraf
Monash Health, Monash University, Melbourne, VIC, Australia

H. Ashraf
Austin Health, Monash University, Melbourne, VIC, Australia

© The Author(s), under exclusive license to Springer Nature
Switzerland AG 2022
M. A. Khan et al. (eds.), *Medical Analogies for Clinician-Patient
Communication*, https://doi.org/10.1007/978-3-030-87293-9_9

73

S. Ashraf · A. Rawal
Monash University, Clayton, VIC, Australia

Y. Hassan
The University of Melbourne, Melbourne, VIC, Australia

I. Ashraf
James Cook University, Douglas, QLD, Australia

Z. Hasimoglu
Latrobe University, Melbourne, VIC, Australia

Contents

HIV and AIDS

Fleas on a Farm

Your body is like a big farm with your various cells being the livestock. The farm is so big that there are hundreds of sheepdogs. Sheepdogs are like your immune cells and they keep your body safe. HIV is like the fleas.

Fleas will first infect the sheepdogs, and they don't even feel that they have been infected. Over time, the fleas overburden and eventually kill the sheepdog. You may not even notice this because there are so many sheepdogs to protect your livestock. Similarly, HIV will infect your immune cells and kill them without showing any signs of it. Slowly, more and more sheepdogs are infected by fleas and die. Eventually, enough sheepdogs get infected by fleas and die that there are only a few sheepdogs left. This makes attacks on your livestock much more likely and much more dangerous. Similarly, HIV will keep infecting and killing immune cells, just like the fleas infect and kill the sheepdogs, until there are only a few immune cells left. Your farm, your body, is then much more susceptible to attacks, such as infections, which can damage it much more severely.

Vaccinations and Autism

Bridge

Imagine a bridge that everyone uses. Very rarely, a car may crash on the bridge. Did the bridge cause the car crash? No, cars go over it day and night. Sometimes in life a car crash occurs, but that doesn't make it the bridge's fault. Similarly, vaccinations have been proven to have no relation with causing autism, just like the bridge didn't cause the car crash.

Just because there was a car crash on the bridge yesterday doesn't mean everyone will stop using the bridge. What is the alternative – swimming in the river below? The risks of the alternative outweigh the necessity of using the bridge.

Flat Tire and Gas

If you put petrol in your car and then later get a flat tire, that doesn't mean that putting petrol in your car caused the flat tire. The two events were merely a coincidence. The same applies for vaccinations and autism.

Vaccinations – Mechanism of Action

Wanted Poster

Vaccines are like a wanted poster; they just show your body what the bad guys look like and how to deal with them. When actually faced with them, your body is prepared and able to stop them before they cause harm.

Social Distancing

Matches

Imagine that every person is like a matchstick. If they are close to one another and one catches fire, they all will. Similarly, if one person has an infection, it is very easy for it to spread if people are close enough. If we spread the matches out far enough, there's very little chance that the lit match will light others. Similarly, if we socially distance, we can stop infected individuals from spreading the infection.

Dominos

If dominos are placed very close together, and one topples, it will cause all of them to fall. However, if you place them far apart, one of them falling won't impact any of the others.

Isolation Period

Tall and Short Candles

Infections are active for different times, just like short and tall candles burn for different times. Tall candles can stay lit for a long time and hence can burn anything close to it for a long time. Similarly, some infections take a long time to stop being infectious, like a tall candle, so we need to isolate for a longer time.

Herd Immunity

Umbrellas

Imagine that a virus is like rain. How do you avoid rain? You could hold an umbrella, which would deflect any rain from wetting your clothes. This is like a vaccine, which is able to help your body deflect an infection from harming you. However, some people can't afford umbrellas, just like how some people cannot get the vaccine. How do we protect these people? The only way is if there were so many people who used umbrellas that a person without an umbrella could be covered by walking under everyone else's umbrella. Similarly, if enough people get vaccinated, the person who cannot get the vaccine will also be protected from the infection.

Hospital-Acquired Infection

Car Wash

Hospitals are like car washes. Although car washes clean dirty cars, sometimes their cleaning equipment can have dirt or stones in it. When another dirty car uses the car wash, it may be affected by the dirt or get scratched by the small stones. Similarly, while the doctors are trying to clear bacteria from patients, those bacteria can contaminate a hospital surface or staff member, and eventually infect another patient.

Tuberculosis (TB)

Termite Infestation

Tuberculosis can be thought of as a termite infestation. Unlike ants, a termite infestation can destroy your house. Similarly, tuberculosis is like the termites of lung infections. It is chronic, requires isolation and strong treatment to eradicate.

Necrotising Fasciitis

Forest Fire

Our body has different layers of tissue. These are like a forest, where there are tree tops at the top, bushes in the middle and then grass which is closest to the ground. Necrotising fasciitis is an infection along one of your body's layers, like a fire on one of the layers of the forest. What happens to this fire? It spreads very quickly across the same level, suppose from bush to bush, and more slowly to the other levels, such as down to the grass or up to the treetops. Similarly, necrotising fasciitis is a fast-moving and devastating infection along the outer layers of your body. We have to use strong antibiotics and will need to cut the infected layers out, just like how one would take away the bushes or trees to stop the spread of the fire.

Killing of Gut Microbiota

Police at a Brawl

Your gut has good bacteria, which help in digesting food. Sometimes, bad bacteria invade your body and we use antibiotics to remove them. However, antibiotics can't differentiate the good and bad bacteria. They are like the police arriving at a brawl – they don't know who started it, but they will take everyone away regardless.

Fever of Unknown Origin

Staring at the Trees, Forgetting the Forest

Sometimes, diseases present in unusual ways, which makes it hard to work out what it is. Imagine standing millimetres away from a tree. All you see is wood. You know it's wood, but you can't tell much else about it. You don't know if it is tall or short, blooming or withering, or whether it is in an orchard or a forest. Similarly, we know there is something causing the fever, but right now we don't know enough to be sure about what it is – for this, we need to look at the whole forest.

Finding the Source of the Fire

Your symptoms tell us that something is wrong, but we can't find the source. It is similar to us being able to see a fire in a forest, but not able to identify what the source of the fire is. We need to do a few more investigations before we can be sure about the source.

Musculoskeletal System 10

Muhammad Azaan Khan, Gizem Ashraf,
Hamza Ashraf, Saad Ashraf,
Yusuf Hassan, Alisha Rawal,
Imaan Ashraf, Qazi Sarem Shahab,
and Zehra Hasimoglu

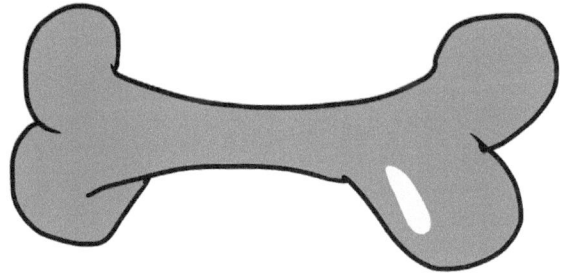

M. A. Khan (✉) · Q. S. Shahab
University of New South Wales, Sydney, NSW, Australia

G. Ashraf
Monash Health, Monash University, Melbourne, VIC, Australia

H. Ashraf
Austin Health, Monash University, Melbourne, VIC, Australia

S. Ashraf · A. Rawal
Monash University, Clayton, VIC, Australia

© The Author(s), under exclusive license to Springer Nature
Switzerland AG 2022
M. A. Khan et al. (eds.), *Medical Analogies for Clinician-Patient
Communication*, https://doi.org/10.1007/978-3-030-87293-9_10

Y. Hassan
The University of Melbourne, Melbourne, VIC, Australia

I. Ashraf
James Cook University, Douglas, QLD, Australia

Z. Hasimoglu
Latrobe University, Melbourne, VIC, Australia

Contents

Bursa

Fluid-Filled Pillow

Think of a bursa like a fluid-filled pillow. It sits between the tendon and bone and acts as a cushion between them.

Carpal Tunnel Syndrome

Cramped Passengers on Train

Imagine carpal tunnel syndrome like passengers cramped on a train. In this syndrome, the nerve running over your arm can be thought of as the trapped passengers. To fix the problem, we need to open the doors and let some people out. Similarly, to treat carpal tunnel syndrome, we can make a small cut and release the pressure inside.

Chronic Osteomyelitis

Archers Attacking a Fortress

Think of osteomyelitis like a fortress. The bacteria builds big walls around your bone. Using antibiotics is like firing arrows at this fortress. You might hit some guards on the edges of the walls, but the arrows can't get to the people inside. To actually solve the problem we need to break down those walls through what we call surgical debridement. Once the wall is broken, we will follow it up with antibiotics. This is like firing arrows at the people inside to get rid of the bacteria.

Fracture

Tree Branches

Imagine your bones as the branches of a tree. They provide support and strength to your body. However, just like sticks, your bones can crack and break. This can range from easy-to-see clean breaks or micro-cracks that are hard to see. Somewhat like branches, given enough time and immobilisation, most fractures will heal themselves without the need for any direct surgical repair.

Gout

Crystallised Sugar in Tea

When you put too much sugar in your tea, it crystallises at the bottom. Similarly, in gout, you have too much 'sugar' or uric acid in your body and the crystals form in small joints such as the ones in your fingers and toes, particularly in the big toe.

Inflammation and Anti-Inflammatories

Massive Storm

Think of inflammation as a big storm which floods a town and causes damage. Some medications (anti-inflammatories), like NSAIDs, will stop the storm.

Non-visualising Fracture

Paper Cut

A non-visualising fracture is like a paper cut. At first it's razor thin and hard to detect, but after a while a scar will develop.

Similarly, we have to wait for a 'scar' to develop in the bone to see it on an X-ray.

Osteoarthritis

Smooth and Jagged Pebbles

Think of a normal joint as rubbing two smooth pebbles together. They easily glide over each other. A joint with osteoarthritis is like rubbing two jagged stones together with the jagged points catching on each other. Similarly, in osteoarthritis, you form small jagged bits of bone and when these 'catch' each other, it causes pain.

Osteoporosis

Termites in a House

Having osteoporosis is like having termites in your house. You don't know they are there until the beams start breaking apart. Similarly, osteoporosis is a 'silent' disease, it doesn't have any symptoms – until you get a fracture.

Paget's Disease of the Bone

Dysfunctional Ant Mound

Bone growth can be visualised as a growing ant mound made by many worker ants. In Paget's disease of the bone, the ant mound is sprayed with pesticide to knock the mound down and kill the worker ants. However, the remaining ants keep trying to rebuild their mound, but this time with less strength. Similarly, Paget's disease of the bone causes bones to be knocked down and rebuilt with poor structural integrity.

Spinal Cord Injury

Highway

Think of the spinal cord as a highway. The multiple lanes are like the multiple nerves running up the cord and the cars on the highway are like nerve impulses. Similarly, there are entrances and exits like those on a highway for nerves to exit. If there is a crash on just one entrance or exit, it's only going to cause problems along that road and the other roads are spared. However, if there's a major crash or a major injury to the spinal cord, it's going to affect multiple roads or nerves. Similarly, if there is a nerve compression at one level, only the function of that particular nerve would be lost. However, if you suffer a transection of the spinal cord, you will damage all the nerves that come off below that level and hence would lose their function.

Sprained Ligament

Tear in a Paper

Imagine a ligament to be similar to a piece of paper. If you hold the paper from either end and pull, nothing happens. But, if you make a tiny rip in the middle and then pull, it will tear. Similarly, spraining your ligament is like making tiny tears and if you pull too hard, you could tear the ligament.

Tendon Rupture

Intertwined Cable

A tendon is like a strong intertwined cable. However, if a tendon ruptures it becomes like a mop – a bunch of shreds.

Torn Meniscus

Hangnail

Think of a torn meniscus like a hangnail on your finger. When it moves around it's painful and it doesn't heal very well. To get rid of it, you can simply clip it off. Similarly, a torn meniscus doesn't heal very well and causes pain on movement and we treat it by going in and clipping off the damaged part.

Nephrology

11

Muhammad Azaan Khan, Gizem Ashraf,
Hamza Ashraf, Saad Ashraf,
Yusuf Hassan, Alisha Rawal,
Imaan Ashraf, Qazi Sarem Shahab,
and Zehra Hasimoglu

Contents

M. A. Khan (✉) · Q. S. Shahab
University of New South Wales, Sydney, NSW, Australia

G. Ashraf
Monash Health, Monash University, Melbourne, VIC, Australia

H. Ashraf
Austin Health, Monash University, Melbourne, VIC, Australia

S. Ashraf · A. Rawal
Monash University, Clayton, VIC, Australia

Y. Hassan
The University of Melbourne, Melbourne, VIC, Australia

I. Ashraf
James Cook University, Douglas, QLD, Australia

Z. Hasimoglu
Latrobe University, Melbourne, VIC, Australia

© The Author(s), under exclusive license to Springer Nature
Switzerland AG 2022
M. A. Khan et al. (eds.), *Medical Analogies for Clinician-Patient
Communication*, https://doi.org/10.1007/978-3-030-87293-9_11

BPH

Straw Through Doughnut

Imagine your prostate is like a doughnut and the urethra is like a big straw going through the hole. When your prostate gets bigger, it starts pressing on the straw. This makes it harder for water to go through the straw. Similarly, in BPH the prostate grows and compresses on the urethra making it difficult to urinate.

BPH Treatment: TURP

Scrape Off Doughnut

We can put a thin tube through the straw and then use that to scrape or burn off the walls of the straw as well as the doughnut so it doesn't squeeze the straw anymore. Similarly, we can scrape or burn off the walls of the urethra as well as the prostate so it doesn't squeeze on the urethra anymore.

Rebore a Metal Cylinder

Imagine your urethra is a metal cylinder which is too narrow. Through a TURP, we rebore it to the right width.

Burning Sensation Post-TURP

Soap on Grazed Skin

When you wash your hands with soap, it doesn't hurt. But if you graze your skin and then wash your hands with soap, it would burn. In a TURP we are taking off the 'skin' of the urethra which means that the soap, or your urine, will now be directly touching your prostate which has been grazed. That's why you might feel a burning sensation when you urinate.

Symptomatic Treatment Before Removing Kidney Stone

Car Crash

An obstruction is like a car crash in the middle of the highway. You need to get the car off the highway and back to safety first, and then you can figure out what went wrong and try to fix it. Similarly, we need to fix your obstruction first with this stent, and then we can deal with the actual problem.

Kidney

Water Treatment Plant

Think of your kidney as a water treatment plant, except that instead of filtering water it filters blood. The waste products plus a bit of water become your urine and the treated water or blood is returned to your blood vessels. If you have a kidney problem, the nephrologists and urologists are like the engineers who figure out what's wrong and treat you.

Kidney Failure

Broken Pool Filter

Let all the blood in your body be represented by a pool filled with water, and your kidneys are the pool filter removing all the waste products. However, if this filter gets broken, suddenly all the toxins build up in the pool, resulting in many unwanted effects. Similarly, your body suffers in multiple ways when your kidneys are failing.

Your kidneys, like a pool filter, can be broken in numerous ways. They can have their energy supply cut off, which is similar to pre-renal causes, resulting in inadequate blood supply. They can be directly damaged, which is similar to renal causes such as toxins or cellular death. They can also be clogged downstream by debris blocking the system's flow, such as post-renal obstruction.

Kidney Dialysis and Transplant

Replacing Pool Filter

Let all the blood in your body be represented by a pool filled with water, and your kidneys are the pool filter removing all the waste products. However, if this filter gets broken, suddenly all the toxins build up in the pool, resulting in many unwanted effects.

Similarly, your body suffers in multiple ways when your kidneys are failing.

In order to correct these adverse effects, we need to somehow remove the waste products, now that our filter is broken. We can do this rather rapidly by hiring a pool cleaner to remove the waste; however, this is only a temporary solution, as waste will continue to build up in the pool over the next few days. Consequently, we will need to hire the pool cleaner every few days to ensure our pool stays waste-free. This is similar to how dialysis works. Since your kidneys aren't removing waste well enough, you will need an external source of waste removal every few days to do the job of the kidneys. No matter how great the initial cleaning is by the pool cleaner, some waste will undoubtedly build up between pool cleaner visits, thus resulting in some lingering adverse effects.

Alternatively, we can permanently keep our pool waste-free by replacing the pool filter altogether. In relation to your kidneys, this is similar to a renal transplant where you receive someone else's kidney.

Kidney Function and Dysfunction

Savings Account in Bank

You can think of your kidneys like the savings account in your bank. At birth, if you are born with two normal kidneys, you have enough 'kidney function savings' to last your entire life. This is as if you had enough savings to provide for you your entire life. As you get older, those savings start to get used up, and this is when problems can start. Eventually, you might have used up all of your savings, which means your kidneys don't function as well, and you can develop kidney disease.

If someone is born with a problem in their kidneys, then this is like starting with less money in your savings account. The money will get used up much quicker, which means you might have kidney problems much earlier on in your life.

If someone goes through a natural disaster they might have to spend lots of money from their savings account to rebuild their house, for example. This is similar to if you had an infection or other illness in your kidney – it may recover (i.e. you may get that money back from the insurance), or it may be permanently damaged and therefore more likely to get damaged in the future, which is why having an acute kidney problem can increase your risk of chronic kidney problems.

Kidney Stones

Choking on Food

Imagine urine flowing through the ureter like drinking water. It flows through quite easily. A stone in your ureter is as if you choked on a big rock – the ureter starts spasming and writhing, which causes intense pain.

Pebble Stuck in Hose

The kidney is like a water tank, the ureter is like a hose coming out of it, and the kidney stone is like a pebble. The pebble isn't an issue if it's in the tank but once it is in the hose it can cause blockage. Similarly, when a kidney stone is in the kidney it usually does not cause an issue but if it moves into the ureter it can cause blockage.

Prostate Cancer

Sloth

Different cancers grow at different speeds. Lung cancer is very aggressive and fast, like a jaguar. But prostate cancer is very slow, like a slow-moving sloth.

Prostate Cancer Screening

Turtle, Rabbit and Leopard

Prostate cancer grows at different rates. Some cancers are like turtles – these will grow very slowly and will actually never cause harm. Other cancers are like leopards – they grow so fast that even if we managed to pick it up early we would not have been able to do anything and the patient would have died of the cancer regardless. In both of these groups, it will not be beneficial to do any screening or treatment because it would not actually change the patient's outcome.

The third group of cancers are like rabbits, who are faster than turtles, so the cancer would impact them, but not too fast like leopards, so we can actually cure them. However, the problem is that even if we screen for prostate cancer, we find out that your cancer is one of these three animals but we don't know which one. This is why prostate cancer screening is no longer recommended. We can screen all the animals, but for every rabbit we save, we are actually harming 40 turtles and leopards and even killing one of them due to the unnecessary investigations we will perform. This harm can be in the form of unnecessary investigations and surgeries (e.g. a turtle got a surgery they never needed) or even just emotional trauma (e.g. a turtle, who would never have known they have prostate cancer, will now live the rest of their life with this fear).

Prostate Cancer Monitoring Post-Diagnosis

Weight Loss

Imagine you're going on a new diet and exercise plan to lose weight. Most weeks you lose a little bit of weight, but some weeks you might not lose any weight and other weeks you may actually gain some weight. However, if you look at the overall trend, you are still losing weight over time, and those 1 or 2 weeks where you gained a little bit of weight don't matter. This is the same with your prostate-specific antigen (PSA) level – a small rise in one or two blood tests doesn't necessarily mean something bad has happened, it is more important to look at the overall trend.

Raised Prostate-Specific Antigen (PSA)

False Fire Alarm

Whenever a fire alarm goes off, we are more likely to think that it's probably an emergency response drill or someone forgetting to turn the stove off, instead of it being an actual fire. However, an alarm going off too often would make one stressed unnecessarily. This is the case with using PSA for prostate cancer screening. PSA can be elevated in a lot of other diseases of the prostate besides prostate cancer, such as benign prostatic hyperplasia (BPH). Therefore, an elevated PSA might put patients through unnecessary tests that come with their own stress and tests that they don't actually need. Therefore, regular PSA level screening is not recommended for prostate cancer.

Stress Incontinence

Spilling Glass of Water

Imagine you're holding a glass of water. If someone came up and scared you, you might get startled and accidentally shake the glass causing some water to spill out. Now think of the glass of water as your bladder, and the person scaring you is an action like coughing or sneezing, and that 'scare' to the bladder makes it spill out a little bit of water, which we call incontinence.

Urethral Stricture

Blocked Pipe

Think of your urethra as a pipe, and over time it gets blocked by the build-up of gunk. We call this build-up 'scarring' and it makes your urethra narrow, therefore making it hard for urine to get through.

Urinary Tract Infection

Road to a Castle

Think of your bladder as a castle which has a road leading to it. If an enemy wants to attack the castle, a shorter road will make it easier for them to reach your castle, whereas a longer road will make it difficult. As females have shorter urethras than males, it is easier for bacteria to get into their bladder. This is why females get UTIs more often than males.

Neurology

12

Muhammad Azaan Khan, Gizem Ashraf,
Hamza Ashraf, Saad Ashraf,
Yusuf Hassan, Alisha Rawal,
Imaan Ashraf, Qazi Sarem Shahab,
and Zehra Hasimoglu

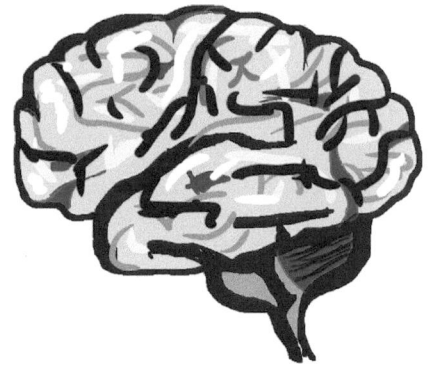

M. A. Khan (✉) · Q. S. Shahab
University of New South Wales, Sydney, NSW, Australia

G. Ashraf
Monash Health, Monash University, Melbourne, VIC, Australia

H. Ashraf
Austin Health, Monash University, Melbourne, VIC, Australia

© The Author(s), under exclusive license to Springer Nature
Switzerland AG 2022
M. A. Khan et al. (eds.), *Medical Analogies for Clinician-Patient
Communication*, https://doi.org/10.1007/978-3-030-87293-9_12

S. Ashraf · A. Rawal
Monash University, Clayton, VIC, Australia

Y. Hassan
The University of Melbourne, Melbourne, VIC, Australia

I. Ashraf
James Cook University, Douglas, QLD, Australia

Z. Hasimoglu
Latrobe University, Melbourne, VIC, Australia

Contents

Blood-Brain Barrier

Moat Around Castle

The blood–brain barrier is like a moat around a castle, which is your brain. It stops harmful things from getting into the castle, and only those things that we want can cross the barrier by putting down the drawbridge and letting them in.

Mass Effect in Brain

Office Departments

Think of your brain like an office floor with many specialised departments, all in their own cubicles. A brain tumour is like one department which randomly starts expanding beyond its cubicle. It takes over the adjacent cubicle and the next; it's unstoppable. As it expands, it disrupts the functions of all those departments it takes over, and can even have distant effects outside the office due to the work disturbances it's causing. Additionally, the office floor has limited space. Hence, the more space the expanding rogue department takes, the more cramped the other departments become, causing damaging effects across the entire office floor. In the same way, a brain tumour can disrupt function within adjacent and distant structures.

Coma, Permanent Vegetative State, and Brain Death

Sleep Mode

Think of your brain as a computer's motherboard, which is in charge of all of its functions. In the event of serious damage, your brain can no longer keep the body running at maximum performance. Instead, like a computer trying to conserve energy, it enters "sleep mode" and shuts down all non-essential systems. When this occurs, it's called a coma. The computer may display a screensaver in this state, which is why you can see some responses like a heartbeat and bowel motions.

A permanent vegetative state is when enough damage to the motherboard has occurred so that no matter how many times you press the 'on' button, the computer never wakes from sleep mode. Brain death is when the computer has lost all ability to turn on again.

Dementia

Filing Cabinet

Think of your brain as a set of filing cabinets. When you want to retrieve some information, you open one filing cabinet and take it out. In dementia, some of those filing cabinets get rusty and hard to open. This means you can't retrieve the information as well as you used to, which is why people with dementia have memory loss. As time goes on, more and more filing cabinets get stuck which is why memory loss worsens. Some dementia medications can unjam the filing cabinets but unfortunately this doesn't always work.

Epilepsy

Whale

Epilepsy can be compared to a whale. You can see the water spout, which is the seizure, but you might not actually see the whale (the cause of the epilepsy) itself. There are times you don't see the whale at all, at other times you can see a little bit, and sometimes it breaches so you can see a lot. Similarly, sometimes we can find the cause of epilepsy but at other times we can't.

Often we don't have anti-whale drugs so we can't treat the cause of the seizures, we only have anti-spout drugs which can stop or improve the symptoms of seizures.

Meningitis

Bubble Wrap

The meninges are the outer covering of the brain. They are like a bubble wrap which protects a package from the outside world. Similarly, the meninges protect the brain from any damage or infection.

However, imagine the air pockets within the bubble wrap get nasty bugs within them that grow and expand the bubble wrap. Now our package is in danger of being squashed by the expanding bubble wrap, or the bugs may pass through the wrapping and infect the package as well. Similarly, meninges which are infected can enlarge and squash the brain, or can go into the blood, which the body then has to fight off.

Multiple Sclerosis

Frayed Electrical Wire

Imagine an electrical wire where the insulation has worn away and the inside wire is exposed, so it short-circuits. This is what happens in multiple sclerosis. The insulation on your nerves, called myelin, has worn away and so the nerves aren't working properly, which causes your symptoms.

Parkinson's Disease

Failing Lightbulb

The area of the brain which controls movement is like a lightbulb. When it is healthy, the lightbulb functions as it is supposed to, turning on and off when required. However, eventually the lightbulb takes longer to turn on, which is similar to Parkinson's patients being slower in their movements. Eventually, the lightbulb can even start to flicker. This is like a tremor, where the muscles shake. Ultimately, the lightbulb can start to lose its light and become dim and eventually turns off, which can be compared to end-stage Parkinson's disease where the movement symptoms are severe and the person can develop dementia.

Peripheral Neuropathy

Walkie-Talkies

Your brain and limbs are constantly in communication, sending information back and forth. We can imagine this communication as a two-way walkie-talkie system. While these walkie-talkies normally have great reception, there can be times when the reception is poor, which makes listening to instructions given by the brain difficult to understand. This may begin with difficulties registering temperature changes or pain, which is like hearing static through the walkie-talkie. Over time, there is more static, which means you progressively lose the function of your limbs, which can be sensory or motor function.

Sciatica

TV Antenna

Sciatica refers to a pattern of pain radiating down the leg due to a disc herniation pressing on and irritating a nerve right next to the spinal cord. This is similar to the old TV antennas that had to be kept in a certain orientation to make sure they were working normally, with small changes to their position leading to poorer image and sound quality. In the same way, we can think of the nerve as an antenna that is also vulnerable to disturbance, like a bit of disc pressing on it, leading to poorer function, including pain and altered feeling and muscle control.

Seizure

Lightning Striking a Building

A seizure is like when lightning hits a building – every single machine in the building gets overloaded with electricity so it malfunctions. When the lightning strike passes, the machines return to normal function. Similarly, a seizure is an electrical overload of the brain, which causes your body to malfunction, causing the symptoms. Once the seizure passes, your body will return to normal function.

Seizure Timing

Ship at Sea

Epileptic seizures often come without warning like a ship being at sea and not knowing when a storm will hit. Sometimes you can notice a change in the weather or see some dark clouds before the storm hits. These warning signals are called an aura.

Stroke

Heart Attack

Every organ needs a good blood supply to survive. But when this supply line is blocked, the part of the organ beyond that blockage dies. This is classically seen in a heart attack, where the blood supply to the heart is blocked. However, this can also happen in the brain, resulting in dead brain tissue if the blood supply isn't restored quickly enough. In a few people, the pipe isn't blocked, it has burst, but the result is still the same dead brain tissue.

Stroke

Household Appliances

In a stroke, a clot blocks the blood vessel causing a part of the brain to die, which can have different effects. It can be compared to when you lose the power supply to an appliance in your house. Sometimes it's your fridge so you can't store food, sometimes it's your phone so you can't call anyone, or your washing machine so you can't do your laundry. Similarly, different strokes affect different parts of the brain and have different effects.

Stroke and Traumatic Brain Injury

Earthquake

Imagine a city is affected by an earthquake which damages buildings, bridges and roads. You might not be able to eat at the local restaurant like you used to or take the same road to work anymore. Similarly, a traumatic brain injury or stroke damages the cells and roads in your brain, so you might not be able to do the same things you used to or you might not be able to do them as well as you used to.

Sometimes, it is possible to rebuild after an earthquake, but at other times the damage is too severe and a building might be lost forever. Similarly, it might be possible to regain some function but at other times there might be little to no improvement, even after many years.

Transient Ischaemic Attack (TIA)

Circuit Trip During a Storm

Imagine there is a big thunderstorm which causes your house to temporarily lose power. The appliances which are affected won't work, but once the thunderstorm has passed the electricity can come back again and the appliances will work. Similarly, a transient ischaemic attack (TIA) causes part of your brain to lose blood temporarily, which means you temporarily might not be able to speak or walk. However, when the TIA resolves, you will gain normal function again.

However, if your appliances have been broken once, it is more likely that they will break a second time. There is also an increased risk that in future times they might break permanently. Similarly, a TIA increases the risk of a future TIA, and also increases the risk of permanent damage, which we call a stroke.

Tension Headache

Paracetamol for a Tension Headache

Taking repeated paracetamol for a tension headache unfortunately isn't the solution. Imagine you had a friend who got a headache because they kept hitting themselves in the head. You wouldn't keep giving them paracetamol, right? You would have to stop the actual problem. Similarly, paracetamol isn't the answer, we need to fix the issues causing the headache, which are the tensions and stressors in your life.

Ophthalmology

13

Muhammad Azaan Khan, Gizem Ashraf,
Hamza Ashraf, Saad Ashraf,
Yusuf Hassan, Alisha Rawal,
Imaan Ashraf, Qazi Sarem Shahab,
and Zehra Hasimoglu

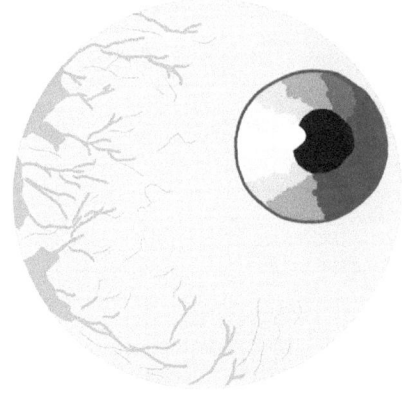

M. A. Khan (✉) · Q. S. Shahab
University of New South Wales, Sydney, NSW, Australia

G. Ashraf
Monash Health, Monash University, Melbourne, VIC, Australia

H. Ashraf
Austin Health, Monash University, Melbourne, VIC, Australia

© The Author(s), under exclusive license to Springer Nature
Switzerland AG 2022
M. A. Khan et al. (eds.), *Medical Analogies for Clinician-Patient
Communication*, https://doi.org/10.1007/978-3-030-87293-9_13

S. Ashraf · A. Rawal
Monash University, Clayton, VIC, Australia

Y. Hassan
The University of Melbourne, Melbourne, VIC, Australia

I. Ashraf
James Cook University, Douglas, QLD, Australia

Z. Hasimoglu
Latrobe University, Melbourne, VIC, Australia

Contents

Astigmatism

Sports Ball Curvatures

Normally, the eyes are meant to be spherical in nature like a basketball, particularly at the cornea which is the clear front of your eye. In someone with astigmatism, the cornea has a non-spherical shape, like a rugby ball. Just like a rugby ball doesn't bounce straight up-and-down like a basketball, your cornea can't focus images correctly like a spherical cornea can.

Blepharitis

Sand

It is an inflammation of your eyelids, which feels like there is sand underneath your eyelid.

Cataract

Glasses Inside the Eye

Just like there are glasses on the outside, everyone has a lens inside of their eyes to help give you a sharp view. With time, glasses can get dirty and scratched, making it hard to see through; eventually they become so bad that we need to replace them. The same is true for the lens inside your eye. Therefore, we have to replace the lens inside your eye to give you a clear view again.

Egg Yolk

The egg white of a raw egg is transparent and you can see through it, but once it is cooked the transparent substance becomes opaque and this is an irreversible change. Similarly, the lens in your eye which was clear has become opaque from aging. This is also an irreversible change. This clouding of your lens, called a cataract, causes your vision to become unclear.

Cataract Surgery

Candy in a Wrapper

The lens sits in a capsule, like a little candy would sit in a wrapper. Imagine the candy is rotten, but we want to keep the wrapper. To do this, we cut a small hole in the wrapper, scoop out the candy, and slide a new candy in there. For you, we cut a small hole in your capsule, break up and scoop out the lens, and put a new lens in there.

Conjunctivitis

Onion Layers

Your eye has layers like an onion. If an onion falls down, it shows a large bruise. Similarly, if your eye becomes infected or responds to allergens, the outer layer, called the conjunctiva, becomes inflamed and red. However, the inner layers of the onion are still fine, just as the inner layers of the eye are unaffected. Unlike a bruised onion, our outer eye layer heals and becomes normal again; we just need to give it time.

Corneal Pathology

Car Windshield

Your cornea is like your car windshield. You would have trouble seeing through your car windshield if it were to get dirty or spotty, just as you are having trouble seeing though your cornea because it is dirty or spotty due to infection or trauma.

Corneal Ulcer

A Meteor Hitting the Earth

The cornea is the clear part of the eye that is in front of the pupil. It allows light to enter and helps us see. Sometimes when the cornea is infected with bacteria, viruses or fungi, an ulcer can form on the cornea. Imagine the eyeball is like the Earth – if a meteor came and hit the earth, a crater would be left behind. This crater on the eyeball is called a corneal ulcer and this can likely cause pain. Individuals wearing contact lenses are at a higher risk of getting corneal ulcers because there may be germs trapped underneath.

Diabetic Retinopathy

Botanical Gardens

Think of your body as a botanical garden with each of the organs being different plants. There are lots of different plants, some that survive with little water and some need water all the time. Your body is also like this, with some organs – like the eyes – needing much more blood than the rest of the body. Just as a botanical garden has water pipes to deliver water, our body has arteries to deliver blood. If the water pipes are leaky and have poor flow, less water will go to the plants and they will be the first to wither and die. The same thing can happen to your arteries from diabetes, therefore making them ineffective in delivering enough blood to your organs. Since your eyes need much blood flow, the poor flow due to diabetes can cause serious effects eventuating in permanent vision loss.

Diabetic Retinopathy – Neovascularisation

Botanical Gardens and Roots

One way the water-hungry plants try to fix the lack of water is to grow roots to suck more water. Your eyes will do the same thing to try to get more blood, where they will make new arteries in the back of your eye. But the problem with these arteries is that they are leaky and break easily, which can permanently damage the eye. Just like we would trim those new roots the water-hungry plants made because they are damaging, we need to stop these arteries from forming.

Dry Eye

Skin Moisturising

Dry eye is like dry skin that needs moisturising. For dry eyes we use lubricating eye drops to moisturise.

Glaucoma

Bathtub

Your eye is filled with nutrient-rich fluid, like a bathtub filled with water. A gland within your eye acts like a faucet and makes this fluid. There is also a drain for the fluid. In glaucoma, you have too much of this fluid in your eye.

In closed-angle glaucoma the drain is blocked by a stopper, so the bathtub overfills very quickly. The eye can't overflow to any other space, so the pressure builds inside and irreversibly damages it.

In open-angle glaucoma the drain has become rusty or grimy, making it less able to drain the fluid efficiently. The eye can't overflow to any other space, so the pressure builds inside it and eventually damages it irreversibly.

To treat this, we can either turn down the faucet or make the drain larger to stop the overflow.

Macular Degeneration

A Clock That Doesn't Tell the Time

The reason we can see things is because of a thin layer of cells lining the back of the eyeball called the retina. If you were to imagine the retina as the size of a small coin, then the macula is a very tiny pinhead-sized oval in the centre of this coin that lets us see things crystal clear. The macula allows us to read the newspaper or make out the facial features of our loved ones when we are looking at them. In macular degeneration, the macula is affected, and this means that our central vision decreases, but the vision in the periphery, or the sides, does not. If someone with macular degeneration were to look at a clock, they would not be able to tell you where the hands of the clock were facing but they might be able to see the numbers around the edges or the rim of the clock and the surrounding wall that the clock is mounted onto.

Optic Neuritis

Electric Wire

The optic nerve is like an electric wire connecting your eyes and brain. In optic neuritis, the covering of the wire becomes inflamed, which impairs the wire's signals. With enough damage to this wire, there can be loss of vision.

Reusing a Daily Contact Lens

Reusing a Dirty Glove

Reusing a daily contact lens is like reusing a one-use dirty glove. It isn't clean even if it looks like it, and can lead to serious infections.

Strabismus

Wheel Misalignment

Just as the wheels of a car are all aligned so the car drives straight, you have eye muscles which help align the eyes to look toward the same place together. Just as a car with misaligned wheels will keep veering to one side, in strabismus, the muscles are not properly aligned, so you can't look directly at something with both eyes. If we don't correct the wheel misalignment, eventually the car's steering system and suspension will become permanently damaged. Similarly, if the eye alignment isn't corrected, there will be irreversible vision loss, which we call amblyopia.

Paediatrics

14

Muhammad Azaan Khan, Gizem Ashraf,
Hamza Ashraf, Saad Ashraf,
Yusuf Hassan, Alisha Rawal,
Imaan Ashraf, Qazi Sarem Shahab,
and Zehra Hasimoglu

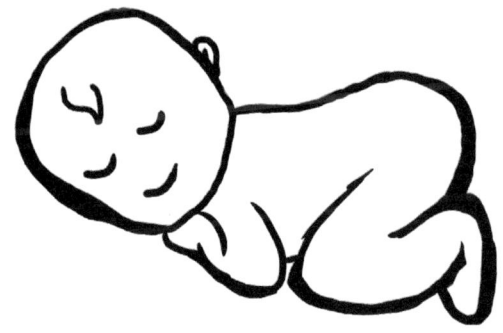

M. A. Khan (✉) · Q. S. Shahab
University of New South Wales, Sydney, NSW, Australia

G. Ashraf
Monash Health, Monash University, Melbourne, VIC, Australia

H. Ashraf
Austin Health, Monash University, Melbourne, VIC, Australia

S. Ashraf · A. Rawal
Monash University, Clayton, VIC, Australia

© The Author(s), under exclusive license to Springer Nature
Switzerland AG 2022
M. A. Khan et al. (eds.), *Medical Analogies for Clinician-Patient
Communication*, https://doi.org/10.1007/978-3-030-87293-9_14

117

Y. Hassan
The University of Melbourne, Melbourne, VIC, Australia

I. Ashraf
James Cook University, Douglas, QLD, Australia

Z. Hasimoglu
Latrobe University, Melbourne, VIC, Australia

Contents

Allergies

Superman and Kryptonite

When you have an allergy, a substance that is harmless to most people can hurt and weaken you even in very small amounts. Just as kryptonite is dangerous for Superman, the allergen can turn out to be very dangerous for you and you need to stay away from it.

Cardiac Septal Defects

Broken Pool Filter

Imagine that the heart is a pool filter and that oxygen is chlorine. The pool filter will pump chlorine-rich water into the pool, and suck up chlorine-deplete water to add chlorine to it before putting it back into the pool. Similarly, in the heart the left-sided chambers collect the oxygen-rich blood from the lungs and send it to all the tissues of the body. The right-sided chambers drain the blood after it has delivered its oxygen and nutrients and send it to the lungs to fill up on oxygen, and then the cycle repeats. In people with normal anatomy, the left chambers never mix with the right chambers, just as how with the pool filter the chlorine-rich water and chlorine-deplete water never mix inside the filter.

Abnormally, some babies are born with an opening between the left side and right sides of the heart. This opening means there is mixing of the oxygen-rich blood and oxygen-poor blood; in a pool filter, this would mean mixing of the chlorine-rich and chlorine-deplete water. If this occurs, the pool will not have properly chlorinated water, so it can't be used correctly. For humans, this means that the blood the body's tissue receives is not completely oxygen-rich, which can suffocate the body's organs and impede growth.

Hirschsprung's Disease

Seaweed Crashing on a Beach

Normally, the muscles in the intestines work together to push faeces through the intestines and anus. Imagine the faeces to be seaweed, and the ocean waves to be the intestine muscles. When a wave forms, it carries the surrounding seaweed with it and tosses it on the beach, just as the intestinal muscles work together to propel faeces through the intestines and anus. However, imagine if the wave suddenly disappeared before reaching the beach. What would happen to the seaweed? It would keep collecting near the coast. Similarly, in Hirschsprung's disease, the propelling wave created by the intestine muscles suddenly stops before the anus, so feces cannot be pushed through the anus, they just remain in the bowel, like the seaweed that never reaches the beach.

Intestinal Atresia

Balloon

Imagine if your intestines were like a long thin balloon. In intestinal atresia, a part of the balloon (intestines) has narrowed. Sometimes this is because the balloon has twisted around itself – like when a clown is shaping a balloon (malrotation with volvulus). At other times, there is a problem with the intestine itself (intrinsic).

Intussusception

Gloves Rolling Back onto Fingers

Think of putting gloves onto your hands. At times, sections of the glove can double roll back onto your fingers. The loops of the bowel can be thought of as these fingers onto which gloves can roll over. Eventually, this results in the sliding of one segment of the bowel onto another (telescoping) which we call intussusception.

Post-Streptococcal Glomerulonephritis

Guard Dog and Thief

A particular bacteria can commonly cause a sore throat or skin infection in children, which resolves after some time. Sometimes however, the body's immune system mistakenly thinks that the bacteria is still in our body and attacks itself – commonly, the kidneys are attacked. Imagine that the immune system is a guard dog of a warehouse, and that the bacteria are thieves. The guard dog will fight the thieves until they are gone, like the immune system fighting the bacteria. Sometime later, the guard dog might mistakenly think that a worker is a thief and fight it. This is similar to the immune system mistaking the kidneys for the bacteria. That worker won't be able to their job, just as the kidneys won't be able to properly do theirs, hence the symptoms in your child.

Jaundice in a Newborn

Water Filling a Bathtub

Jaundice means yellowing of the skin, which results from a build-up of a pigment in the blood called bilirubin. Imagine that the body is a bathtub with the drain unplugged, and that bilirubin is the water pouring from a faucet. Normally, the bathtub has just the right amount. In someone with jaundice, there is too much water in the bathtub, either because the faucet is pouring out too much, or the drain in the bathtub is blocked. Similarly, this means that either the body is producing too much bilirubin, or the body is not able to remove the bilirubin quickly enough. We need to conduct investigations to ascertain the cause and attempt to normalize the bilirubin.

Pyloric Stenosis

Rope Around the Stomach

Just like your body, your stomach also has a neck. Imagine if there was a rope wrapped around your neck compressing your windpipe - it would be hard for air and food to pass through. Similarly, the neck of the stomach, which is in between the stomach and the intestines, also has tissue and muscles surrounding it, called the pylorus. In pyloric stenosis, the tissue becomes very thick, causing it to act like a rope around the stomach. This makes the passage from the stomach to the intestine extremely tight, which leads to regurgitation and vomiting. We can fix this through a surgery where we create more space at the neck so that it is not compressed.

Type 1 Diabetes Mellitus

Vehicles Without Petrol Stations

Imagine that all the different cells in your body are the different types of vehicles on the road: cars, trucks, buses, police wagons, firetrucks, taxis and so on. Every vehicle has a different job, but they all need one thing in common to function: fuel, which they all get through petrol stations. Similarly, all the cells of the body have their own fuel, called glucose or sugar, to function. The petrol station for our bodies is called insulin, and it allows the fuel we eat to reach our cells.

Imagine if the petrol stations were all gone. All the vehicles would stop driving, which would stop them performing their functions. Similarly, in type 1 diabetes, the body's petrol stations, insulin molecules, are all gone. This means that all of the cells of the body can no longer function because of their lack of fuel, just like the vehicles without petrol.

Peri- and Post-Operative Care

15

Muhammad Azaan Khan, Gizem Ashraf,
Hamza Ashraf, Saad Ashraf,
Yusuf Hassan, Alisha Rawal,
Imaan Ashraf, Qazi Sarem Shahab,
and Zehra Hasimoglu

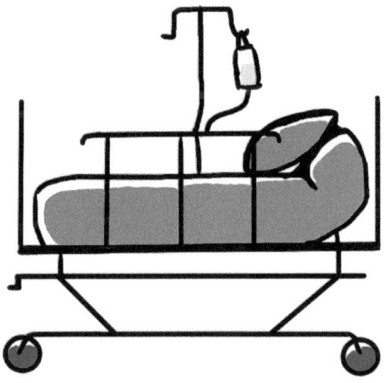

M. A. Khan (✉) · Q. S. Shahab
University of New South Wales, Sydney, NSW, Australia

G. Ashraf
Monash Health, Monash University, Melbourne, VIC, Australia

H. Ashraf
Austin Health, Monash University, Melbourne, VIC, Australia

S. Ashraf · A. Rawal
Monash University, Clayton, VIC, Australia

Y. Hassan
The University of Melbourne, Melbourne, VIC, Australia

I. Ashraf
James Cook University, Douglas, QLD, Australia

Z. Hasimoglu
Latrobe University, Melbourne, VIC, Australia

Contents

Adhesions

Superglue

Adhesions are like bits of superglue in your body. During bowel surgery, your bowel undergoes manipulation, suturing is performed and some sections might be excised, which can trigger an inflammatory response. The inflammation leads to the formation of fibrous bands of tissue. Postoperatively, some sections of the bowel stick together due to the fibrous tissue that is functioning as a "superglue" in this case. These areas of bowel that stick together are known as adhesions. These adhesions can later cause problems with the passage of food boluses and can potentially lead to bowel obstruction.

Electrolyte Imbalances

Bathtub

We can think of electrolyte balance like a filling bathtub. The open tap represents electrolytes going in and the open drain represents electrolytes leaving your body. The water level in the bathtub represents the overall concentration of electrolytes in your blood.

Electrolyte excess: Sometimes the tap might be letting in too much water, which is like when we have too much electrolyte intake.

Electrolyte deficiency: Sometimes the drain may be letting out too much, which is like when we have too much electrolyte excretion.

Electrolytes in cells: The rubber duck is like our cells. Imagine the rubber duck had a hole in it which allowed electrolytes to leak in and out. There are various channels on our cells which allow different electrolytes to flow in and out of our body cells through electrochemical gradients.

Pressure Ulcers

Apples

Stage I: Stage I is like when the apple has a bruise on the outside. Although the skin is intact, patients might have superficial redness.

Stage II: Stage II is like an apple with peeled skin. Patients have partial thickness loss of dermis and present with a shallow open ulcer.

Stage III: Stage III is like an apple that has been bitten into without reaching the core. Patients have full thickness tissue loss. Subcutaneous fat may be visible but bone, tendon and muscle are not exposed.

Stage IV: Stage IV is like a fully eaten apple with only the core left. Patients have full thickness tissue loss with exposed bone, tendon or muscle.

Suspected deep tissue injury: Suspected deep tissue injury is like a bad apple where you can see an external area of bruising and you can feel the inside is soft. Patients have localised area of discoloured intact skin or with damage of underlying soft tissue.

Sepsis

Bushfire

Imagine the human body and its various systems as a big forest. An infection in a particular organ can be compared to a fire starting in one small corner of the forest. It is contained and therefore only directly damaging the local structures. However, as the fire starts to spread it impacts the forest. If we don't intervene immediately, the fire can get out of control and destroy the entire forest. Similarly, if we don't treat sepsis as soon as we recognise it, it can turn out to be a multi-system, life-threatening issue.

The way we treat sepsis is similar to how we manage a bushfire. Initially, we need to support the people trapped in the fire before trying to extinguish the fire. In a patient, this means giving them oxygen and fluids to keep them stable and making sure that their vital organ function is not severely compromised. Secondly, we need to find the source of the infection. In sepsis, this means running various tests to find the source. Thirdly, we need to extinguish the fire. In sepsis, we treat the problem by giving the patient antibiotics. We aim to achieve all of this simultaneously.

Shock

Water Pump and Pipes

Shock is a state wherein different parts of the body do not receive enough blood due to problems with the circulation. It can help us to think about these problems by thinking of a town's water supply. We can either have a problem with the main pumping station (think of the heart), the pipes might have a blockage or we don't have enough water to go around! We give these water problems fancy names starting with cardiogenic, obstructive and hypovolemic shock respectively.

The four types of shock (cardiogenic, distributive, obstructive and hypovolemic) can be thought of in terms of a water pump connected to pipes supplying (the circulatory system) water to homes (end organs). If the pump has problems we have a situation analogous to cardiogenic shock. If the pipes do not have enough fluid in them we get hypovolemic shock. If the pipes enlarge and we have a drop in water pressure, we have something akin to distributive shock (which can be divided into septic and anaphylactic categories). Lastly, if there is a blockage in the pipes we get obstructive shock.

Psychiatry

16

Muhammad Azaan Khan, Gizem Ashraf,
Hamza Ashraf, Saad Ashraf,
Yusuf Hassan, Alisha Rawal,
Imaan Ashraf, Qazi Sarem Shahab,
and Zehra Hasimoglu

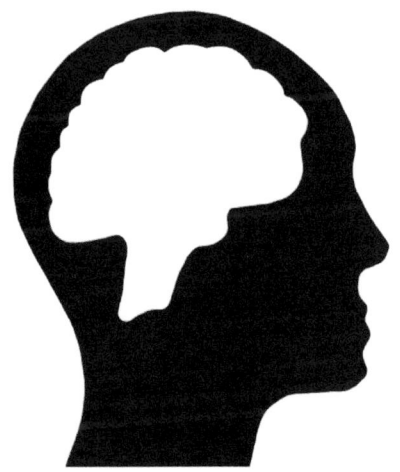

M. A. Khan (✉) · Q. S. Shahab
University of New South Wales, Sydney, NSW, Australia

G. Ashraf
Monash Health, Monash University, Melbourne, VIC, Australia

© The Author(s), under exclusive license to Springer Nature
Switzerland AG 2022
M. A. Khan et al. (eds.), *Medical Analogies for Clinician-Patient
Communication*, https://doi.org/10.1007/978-3-030-87293-9_16

H. Ashraf
Austin Health, Monash University, Melbourne, VIC, Australia

S. Ashraf · A. Rawal
Monash University, Clayton, VIC, Australia

Y. Hassan
The University of Melbourne, Melbourne, VIC, Australia

I. Ashraf
James Cook University, Douglas, QLD, Australia

Z. Hasimoglu
Latrobe University, Melbourne, VIC, Australia

Contents

Addiction

No Brakes

Telling a person with an addiction to 'just quit' is like telling someone driving a car with no breaks to 'just stop'. Although they may want to, they may not have the necessary means. Management is about helping people find brakes that work for them.

Attention Deficit Disorder (ADD)

Computer Tabs

Patients with ADD have difficulty with concentrating on a single task. Their mind is often jumping between thoughts like trying to read a computer screen with lots of tabs open all at once. On top of this, they also get constant pop-up ads that distract them.

Attention Deficit Hyperactivity Disorder (ADHD)

Untuned Radio

Patients with ADHD appear distracted and as though they are not paying attention but it is because they have difficulty concentrating. Concentration for them can be like listening to a radio that isn't tuned in properly. They are only able to catch occasional snippets of information through the static.

Hamster Wheel

Patients with ADHD often use a considerable amount of mental and physical energy. At times they might feel like they are on a hamster wheel that they can't get off.

ADHD Management

Race Car

Patients with ADHD have difficulty with concentration and hyper-activity. Imagine their brain is a race car. Driving a race car safely is not something we can do without practice. Our management of ADHD is aimed at teaching patients how to learn to drive and stay in control of the race car.

Anxiety

Plane with Turbulence

People with anxiety may experience feelings of anxiousness for prolonged periods of time. Most people feel anxious when on a plane with turbulence; however, this usually settles after a few minutes. For people with anxiety, the turbulence on the plane may take longer to settle or not settle at all.

Falling from the Sky

Imagine jumping out of a plane and knowing you will hit the ground but not knowing when it will happen. Similarly, people with anxiety may feel constant fear from waiting for something bad to happen without knowing when.

Bipolar Disease

Tigger and Eeyore (from Winnie the Pooh)

Patients with bipolar disease experience manic and depressive episodes. Manic episodes consist of behaviour like Tigger's inability to sit still, impulsiveness and lack of fear and responsibility. Depressive episodes are like Eeyore's sadness and lack of energy. However, patients with bipolar experience both of these characters or moods.

Weather

Bipolar disease is unpredictable like the weather. Just like you may wake up to a beautiful sunny day and go to bed in a thunderstorm, patients with bipolar disease may have days or weeks of perfect happiness and then experience depression. It's no one's fault when the weather changes, similarly patients don't have full control over their mood.

Bipolar Disease Management

Weather

Just as we have ways of dealing with different weather, for example, a hat on a sunny day or a raincoat on a rainy day, we have different medications to deal with the different moods of bipolar disease. We can use antidepressants for depressive episodes and antipsychotics for manic episodes. We can also use a mood stabiliser. This is similar to an umbrella, which can protect you from the rain but also shield you from the sun.

Distorted Perception

Black Glasses

If you wear black glasses the world will appear black even though it isn't. Similarly, psychiatric illnesses can distort a patient's world view. To complicate things, the patient may not be aware they are wearing glasses which are distorting their world.

Exploring Past History

Finding the Roots

Even though fruit grows on the branches of a tree, we need to water the tree's roots for the fruits to grow. It would not make sense to water the branches. Similarly, sometimes therapy needs to find where the problem stems from and focus on this root cause to find the right solution.

Generalised Anxiety Disorder

Piglet (from Winnie the Pooh)

Patients with generalised anxiety disorder may experience symptoms similar to Piglet's personality. For example, Piglet is afraid of everything, overly nervous and has low self-esteem. Some patients also have difficulty in speaking to others, similar to Piglet's stutter, or have nervous physical habits similar to Piglet's ear twitch.

Magnified Pain

Mind as a Speaker System

Currently I am speaking in a normal voice, but if I were to use a microphone my voice would be amplified. Similarly, sometimes our minds act as speakers and can distort normal experiences to be interpreted as more painful than usual.

Mania

Rollercoaster

Mania is like impulsively going on a rollercoaster ride. During manic episodes patients experience the thrill and excitement of going up high; however, it is only once they are at the top that the manic episode ends and they realise the consequences of their impulsive actions. They then have to deal with the reality of coming down. This involves facing the consequences of their actions and experiencing the drastic downward change in their mood and energy levels.

Messy Filing Cabinet

Your mind is like a file cabinet where all your thoughts and memories are filed neatly away in file folders. Most of the time, everything is neatly ordered and therefore easily accessible. Imagine if all at once those neat files are thrown into disarray and chaos. Suddenly you have no control over which file is in front of you and you are reading through them as fast as you can (pressured speech). Additionally, some files from your imagination, which normally make no sense, are misfiled into reality; you become convinced that they are now real and very significant, which we call delusions.

Normal Investigation Results

Wires and Electric Current

If a light bulb stops working this may be due to a problem with the wires or the electricity. Similarly, problems in our bodies may be due to neurons (wires) or the chemicals they use to communicate (electricity). Most medical tests check for problems with the wires, for example by photographing them (neuroimaging). Since mental illnesses are often related to chemicals they may not be seen in medical tests.

Obsessive-Compulsive Disorder (OCD)

Broken Smoke Detector

Patients with OCD have excessive intrusive thoughts (obsessions) that lead to repetitive behaviors (compulsions). These obsessions may be compared to a broken smoke detector that is regularly beeping to alert you of a danger when there is actually no danger present. Although you know the smoke detector is broken, you still feel the need to act in response to the alert.

Classroom

The mind of a patient with OCD is similar to a classroom. Different students are like different thoughts. Most of the students are quiet and do their work as expected. However, one student is really loud and disruptive (obsessions). This causes another student to become infuriated and react to them angrily (compulsion). The other student must react to the loud student, just as compulsions are a reaction to the obsessions.

Panic Attack

Drowning

Some patients describe their panic attacks to feel like drowning. Initially they are able to hold their breath underwater but when they want to come up for air, they can't get their head above water. The more they panic and struggle, the harder it becomes to breathe.

Same Diagnosis, Different Management

People

If we look at different people, they have the same body parts but are slightly different. For example, they can have different coloured eyes or different hair lengths, even though they are all humans. Similarly, the same condition can be experienced differently and therefore need different treatment and medications.

Therapy

Riding a Bike

We all learn to ride a bike in an empty open space before we enter busy streets with traffic. Similarly, therapy helps develop your skills in a comfortable setting before relying on these skills in stressful situations.

Unintentional Behaviour

Intentional Versus Accidental Kick

Sometimes we find it difficult to tolerate a patient's behaviour. For example, if you are sitting at the cinema and a healthy, alert adult purposefully kicks your seat you would probably be upset. But if the person who kicked you was having an unintentional seizure, you probably wouldn't react the same way. Similarly, some of the patient's behaviours are part of their illness rather than being done on purpose to upset you.

Respiratory

17

Muhammad Azaan Khan, Gizem Ashraf,
Hamza Ashraf, Saad Ashraf,
Yusuf Hassan, Alisha Rawal,
Imaan Ashraf, Qazi Sarem Shahab,
and Zehra Hasimoglu

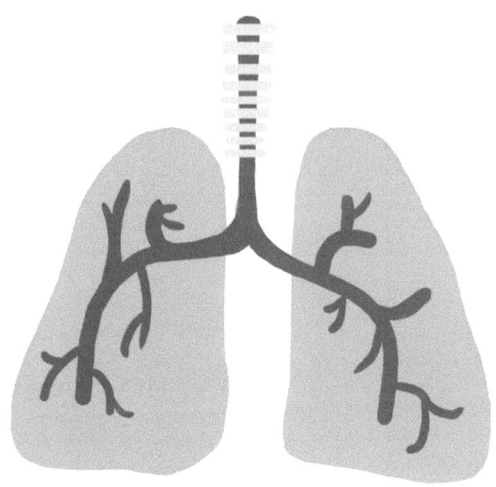

M. A. Khan (✉) · Q. S. Shahab
University of New South Wales, Sydney, NSW, Australia

G. Ashraf
Monash Health, Monash University, Melbourne, VIC, Australia

© The Author(s), under exclusive license to Springer Nature
Switzerland AG 2022
M. A. Khan et al. (eds.), *Medical Analogies for Clinician-Patient
Communication*, https://doi.org/10.1007/978-3-030-87293-9_17

H. Ashraf
Austin Health, Monash University, Melbourne, VIC, Australia

S. Ashraf · A. Rawal
Monash University, Clayton, VIC, Australia

Y. Hassan
The University of Melbourne, Melbourne, VIC, Australia

I. Ashraf
James Cook University, Douglas, QLD, Australia

Z. Hasimoglu
Latrobe University, Melbourne, VIC, Australia

Contents

Airflow Obstruction

Cars on Highway

Think of your airway as a five-lane highway with plenty of space for cars. When there is an obstruction, that same highway now only has one or two lanes, but the same number of cars trying to get through. Similarly, when your airway becomes obstructed, it becomes narrow. The same amount of air is trying to get through, but it can't. This is why it can be difficult to breathe.

Anaphylaxis

Superman and Kryptonite

When you have anaphylaxis, even very small amounts of a substance that is harmless to most people can potentially trigger a life-threatening episode of cardiorespiratory dysfunction. Just as kryptonite is dangerous for Superman, the allergen is dangerous for you so you need to stay away from it.

Antibiotics for a Viral Infection

Broken-Down Car

Using antibiotics for viruses is like putting more fuel in your car when it's actually the battery that's dead – it won't fix the problem.

Asthma – Pathophysiology

Hose

Think of your airways as a hose. Normally water flows freely through a hose, just like air flows freely in your lungs. In asthma, two things happen: initially, the hose gets clogged up with gunk, which represents the inflammation inside the airway. Secondly, the hose wall constricts as if you were squeezing it, which represents the spasm of the airway wall.

Now to treat asthma, we mainly use two medications, ventolin and steroids. Continuing the hose analogy, ventolin immediately stops the squeezing/spasming of the hose wall. This makes it easier for water/air to pass through. The steroids act over a longer period of time to make sure that the hose doesn't get clogged up, which allows the air to flow through smoothly.

Sandcastle on the Beach

The chronic inflammation of asthma comes in waves, like on a beach. Each time the wave comes in and destroys a bit of the sandcastle, you can repair it. But over time, you get tired of rebuilding.

Then, when a strong tide hits, the sand castle is broken beyond repair. This is similar to asthma – we can reverse the initial damage to the airways, but eventually the damage will get so bad that the body gets exhausted after repairing it over and over again. This causes irreversible damage.

Asthma – Treatment

Car Crash

Think of your steroid inhaler as a seatbelt. It is a preventative measure to save passengers from injuries in the case of a crash. Similarly, you need to take your inhaler every day as a preventer.

Your ventolin is known as an asthma reliever. Its role can be compared to that of an airbag. So if you're ever in a car crash or in this case, an asthma attack, the airbag goes to work and protects further injury.

Guard Dogs and Fence

Picture a building protected by a fence, and inside the fence are guard dogs. Now if someone tries to rob the building, usually the fence will stop them. But let's say they do manage to get over the fence, then the guard dogs step in and protect the building.

Your steroid inhaler is like that fence. It makes it much harder for an intruder – which is like an asthma attack – to get into the building. Your reliever is like the guard dogs – it jumps into action if an asthma attack happens, or in the analogy, if an intruder gets past the fence. You don't want your guard dogs barking all the time; similarly, you don't want to be using your reliever on a daily basis since this indicates a weak fence, which means a poorly working preventer.

Atelectasis

Car Tyre

Although your lungs work as two large structures, within them they each have multiple lobes and sacs. You can think of these different areas as different tyres of a car. For the car to function properly all the tyres should be filled with air. Similarly, your lungs have optimum function when all the lobes are able to fill up with air. However, just as a car tyre can become flat, a lobe of your lung can also collapse. When part of your lung collapses we call this atelectasis. The bigger the hole in your car tyre the harder it will be to drive your car. If your tyre is completely flat then it's even more difficult and dangerous. Similarly, if a part of your lung collapses, it is harder for you to breathe. If your entire lung collapses, your risk of developing an infection or respiratory failure increases considerably.

Bronchiectasis

Clothes Stretching Over Time

Bronchiectasis refers to irreversible dilation of your airways after chronic inflammation. This is like wearing clothes which stretch over time as you continue to gain weight – even if you eventually lose weight, the clothes have been irreversibly stretched and damaged.

Bronchitis versus Pneumonia

Respiratory Tree

Think of your respiratory system as a tree. The trunk is your big airways, while the small branches and leaves represent your smaller airways and alveoli. An infection in your big airways is called bronchitis, which is different to an infection in the leaves or alveoli, which is called pneumonia.

Chronic Obstructive Pulmonary Disease (COPD) – Pathophysiology

Balloons Versus Paper Bags

Think of normal lungs as balloons: when you inflate them, they fill up, and when you let the air out, the balloon goes back to its original shape. Lungs in COPD can be compared to paper bags into which air is blown. The bags will fill up if you blow air into it, but when you open the bag not much air comes out and there's still a lot left in the bag.

Cystic Fibrosis (CF)

Breathing Through a Straw

For someone with CF, the airways are blocked with excessive mucus production. It can feel as though one is breathing through a narrow straw. With the progression of the disease, a larger area of the straw gets clogged up with mucous and it gets harder to breathe. This is why patients with CF need to take medications and do lung exercises to clean out the straw every day.

Chewing Food

As adults, we are able to chew our food and swallow it, which allows it to be digested. However, young children may be unable to chew their food, which is why their parents may need to help them, for example by breaking the food into little pieces. Similarly, our gut needs enzymes to break down the food before digesting it. However, in CF the ducts through which these enzymes are released are blocked, which means that the food cannot be digested. Just as children need something external to break down the food for them, people with CF need to take synthetic enzymes which will break down food so that it can be digested.

Brushing a Horse

You brush a horse to clean its mane and remove unwanted particles. Similarly, your lungs have a brush which cleans your airways, called the mucociliary escalator. In CF, this brush stops working properly. Hence, it is difficult for the body to clean the airway. For the horse without a brush, the only way to fix the mane is through constant maintenance and if you don't do this, the horse's mane will easily tangle up and be ruined. Similarly, we have to repeatedly use medications and exercises to help the airways remain clear and clean.

Hole in a Boat

Clogged up airways in CF is like a boat with a hole which is filling with water. At the start, there's little water in the boat so you can bail it out easily, but if you leave it too long it can overwhelm the boat. Similarly, CF management needs to be consistent and daily to be able to clear the mucus-filled airways.

Emphysema

Pens in a Farm

Your healthy lung is like a farm with several pens for livestock; all the pens are made with and connected to each other with wire fencing, which is the alveoli where oxygen mixes with your blood. The more pens we have, the more animals we can put there without them fighting one another.

In a lung with emphysema, all the fences have been knocked down. You may think that you now have more farmland. However, with each fence that was knocked down, there is less room for the animals since they will fight each other for the same food and space. Similarly, in emphysema, your pens, your alveoli, have been knocked down so there is less area for air exchange to occur.

Each cigarette you smoke is like a wirecutter into a fence, which initially just leaves cracks which you might not notice, but which eventually may cause the wall to crumble. Each year you smoke, you knock down one fence in your lung. Each cigarette you give up allows the fences to repair a little, but once the fence, your alveoli, has crumbled it is in the non-reversible stage of the disease.

Broken Wired Fence

Picture a wire fence. Normally, it does its job and you can't get through because the holes are too small. But if every day you cut off some of the wires, eventually the holes would become bigger and you will be able to get through. Soon the fence isn't very useful because the holes are big enough for something to go through. Your alveoli are normally like those little holes. There are a lot of them and they do their job. In emphysema, the walls between alveoli start to break down – just like cutting wires in the fence – eventually, the alveoli aren't very useful.

Heart Failure and Pulmonary Oedema

Overfilling a Glass of Water

In your lungs you have sacs of air which are surrounded by blood vessels. In heart failure, there's too much fluid in those vessels so it starts spilling out into your lungs. This is like overfilling a glass of water – it'll spill onto the ground. When the fluid starts accumulating in your air sacs, it's hard for gas exchange to occur between the blood and the air in the alveoli. This is why you feel short of breath.

Obstructive Sleep Apnoea (OSA)

Plastic versus Paper Straw

When you are awake and breathing, the muscles surrounding your airways are stiff like a plastic straw. However, when you sleep these muscles relax and your airways are more collapsible like a paper straw. Imagine trying to drink a milkshake with a plastic straw. It's quite easy. Similarly, during the day when your airway is stiffer, air can enter and leave your lungs easily. Now, imagine trying to drink a milkshake out of a flimsy paper straw. As you suck in, the paper straw collapses and you don't get any milkshake. This collapsing is what happens to people with OSA but instead of missing out on a milkshake they don't get enough air into their lungs.

Peak Flow Meter

Car Speedometer

Think of the peak flow meter like your car's speedometer – it measures speed. Similarly, the peak flow meter measures how fast the air moves out of your lungs.

Pleural Effusion

Bear Hug

A pleural effusion is a collection of fluid that compresses your lungs from their outer surface. Think of a pleural effusion like someone giving you a bear hug. They wrap their arms around your chest really tightly which makes it hard to breathe because your lungs can't expand.

Pneumothorax

Simple Pneumothorax – Fence Gate

Your lungs are enclosed in a sac which doesn't allow anything inside. A pneumothorax is a tear of this protective sac. Imagine the sac to be a fence keeping out sheep and the tear to be a fault in the gate which allows a few brave sheep through before closing. Instead of sheep, some air has managed to sneak in before the tear closes in your protective sac, but this goes away soon with minimal treatment.

Tension Pneumothorax – Fence Gate

Your lungs are enclosed in a sac which doesn't allow anything inside. A pneumothorax is a tear of this protective sac. Imagine the sac to be a fence keeping out sheep and the tear to be a break in the fencing. The sheep will push through this tear in the fence and eventually they will overcrowd your fenced land. The tear in the fence is such that its easy for the sheep to enter, but impossible for them to leave, like a one-way road. In your example, the tear of your lungs protective sac is like this one-way road. Instead of sheep, it is air that is entering the protective sac, but unable to leave. If we don't fix the tear in the fence, in your pleural sac, then your lungs and heart will be squashed from all the air pushed in and you can go into cardiorespiratory failure.

Pulmonary Hypertension and Cor Pulmonale

Bodybuilder and Heavy Weights

Think of your heart as a bodybuilder. When bodybuilders lift weights they will build muscle, but if you lift weights that are too heavy and for too long, you start getting tired and break down. This can be used to understand heart failure from pulmonary hypertension. If the pressure in the vessels of the lungs is too high, that is, the 'weights' are too heavy, at first your heart just gets bigger and stronger to accommodate this increased pressure, but eventually it can't keep up and you can develop heart failure.

Respiratory Tree and Smoking

Trees, Branches and Leaves

Think of your lungs as an upside-down tree: your trachea is the main tree trunk, then the trachea branches into smaller and smaller airways (called bronchi and bronchioles) like a tree does. Finally, at the end you have the leaves or alveoli. This is where gas exchange takes place, similar to how photosynthesis happens in the leaves.

Think of the effects of smoking on your lungs as burning leaves with a lighter. Over time you'll damage the leaves and they won't be able to do photosynthesis, or in the lung's case, gas exchange, properly.

Tuberculosis (TB)

Spies

TB has three phases: a primary infection, a latent phase – where it is hidden – and a reactivation phase. In this way, it is like a spy from an enemy country. They may activate a few alarms at customs on first arrival, but most spies pass customs. This is like the primary infection, which may exhibit some symptoms or none at all. The spy will then assimilate and work their way into government without anyone noticing. This is the latent phase. When security is busy or relaxed, the spy strikes, causing major damage to your country. This is the reactivation phase, which occurs when your security, your immune system, is weakened due to other health problems.

Like the spy travelled by air to reach your country, TB travels by air and hence starts off in your lungs. Eventually, it can spread all over your body.

Rheumatology

18

Muhammad Azaan Khan, Gizem Ashraf,
Hamza Ashraf, Saad Ashraf,
Yusuf Hassan, Alisha Rawal,
Imaan Ashraf, Qazi Sarem Shahab,
and Zehra Hasimoglu

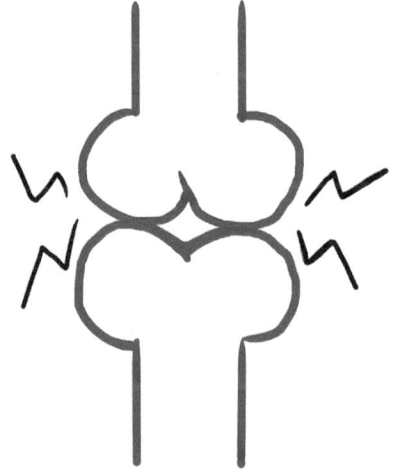

M. A. Khan (✉) · Q. S. Shahab
University of New South Wales, Sydney, NSW, Australia

G. Ashraf
Monash Health, Monash University, Melbourne, VIC, Australia

153

H. Ashraf
Austin Health, Monash University, Melbourne, VIC, Australia

S. Ashraf · A. Rawal
Monash University, Clayton, VIC, Australia

Y. Hassan
The University of Melbourne, Melbourne, VIC, Australia

I. Ashraf
James Cook University, Douglas, QLD, Australia

Z. Hasimoglu
Latrobe University, Melbourne, VIC, Australia

Contents

Autoimmune Disease

Double Agents and Guard Dogs

Your body has inflammatory cells and antibodies, which are like soldiers and guard dogs that protect you from attacks. Most of the time the soldiers and dogs are great at knowing what cells belong to you and what don't. But sometimes they are tricked into believing that some of your body's cells are double agents and so hunt and kill them. We don't know why the soldiers and dogs get so jumpy, but we do know that certain things can make them more jumpy and likely to attack you.

This problem also makes it hard to treat the disease, because you are fighting against your own soldiers and guard dogs, who also protect you from a lot of harmful things. If we get rid of all of your protectors then a serious attack from an outside threat is very likely. If we don't control your protectors at all then they will continue attacking you from the inside.

Fire Sprinkler System

Your immune system in your body is like a water sprinkler system in an office. It is great for putting out fires whenever they occur. But in some buildings there is a false alarm where the sensors think there is a fire when there isn't one, causing the sprinklers to go off. This drenches the whole office, ruining important files and computers. This is what has happened to you. Your immune system has triggered a false alarm because it thinks that there is a fire inside a certain part of your body and so it tries to kill it, which damages your body and causes your symptoms.

Disease-Modifying Anti-Rheumatic Drugs (DMARDs)

Unsafe Car Factory

Our body produces cells all the time using substances we eat, including folic acid found in leafy greens. This is similar to a car-manufacturing factory which receives metal and tyres to build cars. Now imagine if there was a corrupt car company building unsafe cars. Your body is doing the same, making unsafe cells which are hurting you. We can address this problem with a drug called methotrexate. If we take away those tyres and metal, then the unsafe cars cannot be built. Similarly, methotrexate takes away folic acid so the unsafe cells can't be made and harm you. However, taking away materials can have other negative effects on other parts of the body, which explains the side effects of methotrexate.

Gout

Sugar in Tea

When you put too much sugar in your tea, it crystallises at the bottom. Gout is a similar pathological process occurring in your body, but instead of the sugar, it is uric acid making crystals in your big toe.

Excess Banana Peels

When you are eating a fruit like a banana, the leftover waste is the skin. Similarly, your body uses substances called purines, which have a leftover waste called uric acid. Normally when you eat bananas you throw the skin in the bin straight away. Similarly, your body gets rid of the uric acid straight away. But sometimes what can happen is that there is too much of the waste product uric acid. This would be like if you ate a lot of bananas and just threw the skin all over the floor instead of in the rubbish bin. You will walk around your house until one day it gets bad enough that you slip and fall, which causes pain. This is similar to what has happened here. The waste product, uric acid, has kept building up until it has gotten bad enough to cause pain. We first need to deal with the acute issue, which is cleaning up the excess waste of banana peels (uric acid). After that we can make sure you aren't eating too many bananas or you are putting the banana peels in the trash properly, which is analogous to reducing your purine intake or enhancing your uric acid excretion.

Paget's Disease of Bone

Hyperactive Dog Digging Holes in Your Backyard

Your bones experience very tiny dents and fractures all the time from moving and exercise. We don't notice it because whenever this happens, our body quickly makes more bone to patch it up. This is similar to your pet dog who keeps on digging holes in your backyard and you keep trying to fill them. In some people, there is an abnormality in this bone recycling process. The remodelled bone is structurally disorganised and functionally impaired. This can be compared to your dog digging the backyard. If that dog becomes extremely hyperactive and keeps on digging, you would be running around shovelling dirt everywhere without any rest. Eventually, your whole backyard would be a tattered mess. Your bones are like this backyard, which means they are really weak and it is easy for them to break.

Rheumatoid Arthritis

Baby Gums

The bones of your joints are capped with a smooth surface called a synovium which allows bones to slide smoothly against each other so the joint can move. This synovium is like the gums of a newborn, meaning they can slide past each other easily. When you have rheumatoid arthritis, this synovium becomes inflamed. An inflammatory process begins in the synovium which can lead to accumulation of excessive fluid. When the baby starts growing teeth, it becomes harder for its gums to slide smoothly. If the baby slides their jaw side to side now, it will be rough. This is what is happening to your bones. The smooth covering of the bone (synovium) has become rough and every time you move it is painful as you are slowly grinding your bones down.

Car Tyres

We have smooth car tyres so that we can drive smoothly and quickly. Similarly, our bones also have a smooth surface which allows them to slide and move quickly – this surface is called the synovium. If tyres were uneven and rough, then the car ride would be bumpy and it would hurt as we drove. What has happened is that the smooth surface between your bones has become rough and uneven from inflammation which causes the pain. These bad tyres can also damage the suspension in the car and damage the shaft. Similarly, your inflamed synovium is damaging your bones, muscles and ligaments, which can lead to further deterioration if left without treatment.

Sjogren's Syndrome

Closed Taps

Sjogren's syndrome can be compared to a situation where all the taps in your house have been broken so you can't get any water. In this disorder, it is hard to make tears or saliva since the taps, the glands responsible for making tears and saliva, are destroyed by an autoimmune process. We focus on fixing your symptoms of dry eyes and dry mouth with external sources such as medications and eye drops. Immunosuppressive drugs are used to limit the autoimmune process, which is the actual culprit behind the condition.

Systemic Lupus Erythematosus (SLE)

Puppy in a House

SLE damages the body a lot like a new puppy in the house. You never know which part of the house they are going to chew or damage. Different people can have the same breed of puppy, but one might be very docile and harmless, while another just likes chewing the couches and pillows, and a third rips the entire house apart. Similarly, different people with SLE can have different severity of presentations affecting different parts of the body.

Women's Health

Muhammad Azaan Khan, Gizem Ashraf,
Hamza Ashraf, Saad Ashraf,
Yusuf Hassan, Alisha Rawal,
Imaan Ashraf, Qazi Sarem Shahab,
and Zehra Hasimoglu

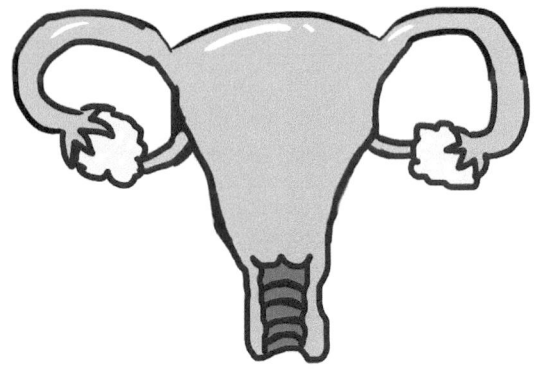

M. A. Khan (✉) · Q. S. Shahab
University of New South Wales, Sydney, NSW, Australia

G. Ashraf
Monash Health, Monash University, Melbourne, VIC, Australia

H. Ashraf
Austin Health, Monash University, Melbourne, VIC, Australia

S. Ashraf · A. Rawal
Monash University, Clayton, VIC, Australia

Y. Hassan
The University of Melbourne, Melbourne, VIC, Australia

I. Ashraf
James Cook University, Douglas, QLD, Australia

Z. Hasimoglu
Latrobe University, Melbourne, VIC, Australia

Contents

Antenatal Testing – Chorionic Villus Sampling Versus Amniocentesis

Egg in Water

Imagine your womb as a pot of water that contains a cracked egg. In the water you have the egg components – the egg white and the egg yolk attached to each other. In this example, the water is your amniotic fluid, the egg white is your placenta and the yolk is your growing baby.

In both chorionic villus sampling (CVS) and amniocentesis, we try to find some of the yolk's cells in the pot without actually touching the yolk. In amniocentesis, we take some of the water; in CVS, we take some of the egg white. This works because we expect some little bits of yolk to have escaped into the egg white and into the water.

As you can imagine, it is slightly more risky poking the egg white. However, the risk of miscarriage is still very low. The amount of water is too low at earlier stages of the pregnancy to take a sample, so we can perform CVS at an earlier time in the pregnancy compared to amniocentesis.

Anti-D Antibody

Identification Markers

Each of your body's cells is marked by your own ID markers. Babies have their own ID markers, separate to their mothers. During pregnancy, there is a specific marker that we worry about called the rhesus marker – you either have it or you don't. For mothers who don't have it, like yourself, we need to be careful if your baby does have it and put in some extra precautions during the pregnancy.

Your cells' ID markers are scanned by your body. If your body recognises them, then it does not attack the cells. However, if it sees something foreign and can't detect your ID marker, it will attack. Your baby has an ID marker that your body has never seen before.

In pregnancy, your baby is safe because your womb hides the baby from the body's ID scanner. But sometimes (during procedures or labour), there is a breach of this safety barrier and some of your baby's cells enter into your body's scanning range. Your body will recognise these cells as foreign and start preparing its defences. We can block this defence by giving you a series of injections that mop up any of the baby's foreign ID markers before your body detects them.

Breast Examination

Bowl of Oatmeal

Think of the breast like a bowl of oatmeal – some lumpiness or even little berries can be expected and are normal. The problem is when there are some hard bits, like a stone disguised as a berry or things stuck to the bowl.

Cervical Dysplasia

Journey on a Long Road

Think of the development of cervical cancer like a long road. The first part of the journey is the development of abnormal changes in the cells of your cervix. The end destination is cancer of the cervix. There are many stages along the way and you can turn back at many points of the road. When you have tests done, we find out how far along the road you have come. When you have a treatment, you take your car back to the start of the road. Most people take between 10 and 15 years before they embark on the risky part of the journey and we can stop their journey before they get there.

Cervical Dysplasia – Understanding Human Papillomavirus (HPV)

Car on the Journey

The most common way for the cells to embark on the journey to cancer is on the HPV car. If we can detect the car on the road then we can stop it from moving along any further. However, if we don't do any screening, then we won't know where any of the cars are along the road and won't be able to treat them.

HPV Subtypes – Different Types of Cars

There are different types of cars – some of them take the cells on the road to cancer and others do not. We are looking for specific cars we know commonly take this road (HPV subtypes 16 and 18) and will investigate them further to check that they are not taking the cells on the road to cancer. The other types of cars we are not as worried about (HPV subtypes besides 16 or 18), but will check them again in a year to make sure they aren't now taking the wrong road.

Fibroids in Pregnancy

Stone in the Soil

The lining of the uterus is where a fertilised egg normally inserts to grow into a foetus. This occurs once sperm has entered the uterus to combine with the egg. This is similar to how seeds in the ground require water from the surface to seep down and help the seed flourish and grow. However, if the water is unable to diffuse down due to a large stone in the ground, the fertilisation and growth of the seed would be hindered. This stone is just like a fibroid which can prevent sperm from entering the uterus and therefore impair the fertilisation of egg. Ultimately, this may contribute to infertility.

Gestational Diabetes Mellitus

Sugar Factory

Diabetes is a condition in which your body cannot control sugar. Normally, a hormone called insulin maintains strict control of your sugar levels. Insulin is like a sugar factory. It controls how much sugar is released into the blood. In diabetes there is a problem with the sugar factory.

In gestational diabetes mellitus (GDM), your womb produces hormones which prevent the factory from working, causing you to lose control of the sugar levels in your body. The factory will hopefully go back to working normally after the pregnancy is over. However, sometimes it remains damaged even after you have given birth.

To keep you and your baby safe, there are a few things we can do to support the factory. Whilst insulin controls the levels of sugar in your blood, we can try controlling how much sugar goes into your body in the first place so that the factory has less work to do. This is firstly through diet, and then some medications that help keep the sugar levels low in your blood. Finally, if none of this works, we can also give you insulin through an injection to do the work of your body's own insulin.

Menopause

Factory

The ovary is like a factory that produces different hormones for your body. In menopause, this factory shuts down. As the factory gets closer to its closing date, the production of the hormones it produces slowly decreases and this has a number of effects on your body. When treating these symptoms, we can import the products from elsewhere by giving you hormone replacement therapy which are synthetic hormones for a short time to restore the balance whilst your body gets used to the factory's closure.

Polycystic Ovarian Syndrome (PCOS)

Factories

The ovaries are like two factories in the city that is your body. In polycystic ovarian syndrome (PCOS), the factories are now malfunctioning and going into overdrive. Whilst they usually produce hormones, the factory is now making more hormones than needed, causing unwanted effects in the city. The excess hormone causes extra hair growth and acne in your body. Normally, when the ovaries take a break is when you get a period. Since the factories are in overdrive, you may also experience fewer or no periods. Because the factories are malfunctioning, they may not complete some of their important jobs – this explains why you may experience a degree of infertility since the ovaries play an important role in fertility.

Prolapse

Pelvic Floor as a Bag

Imagine a bag that you may have used for decades: there are likely to be points in the bag which are weaker than others. Eventually the seams may weaken and things may stick out of your bag. Similarly, the pelvic floor can weaken over time, causing your pelvic organs to protrude and prolapse.

Boat on the Dock

Think of your pelvic organs as a boat on the dock. The boat is held to the dock with ropes (pelvic ligaments) and is sitting on the water below (pelvic floor muscles).

If the water level drops, the ropes may eventually break causing the boat to go down. This is what happens when your pelvic floor muscles weaken and your pelvic organs are no longer supported by the ligaments.

We can fix the ropes, but without the sea level coming back to right level, the boat will still be at risk of falling. If you increase the weight on the boat, or your body, it will fall faster. The best way to stop the boat from falling is to fix the ropes, bring the water level back up and to avoid unnecessary pressure on the boat. That is, to fix the pelvic ligaments and strengthen the pelvic floor muscles below through pelvic floor exercises and reduce the load on it through weight control.

Stress Incontinence

Balloon

Think of your bladder as a balloon filled with air. You are holding the end of the balloon to stop any air coming out but eventually your fingers will get tired. If someone comes and squeezes the balloon, your fingers are not holding the balloon strongly enough and some air will escape. Similarly, in stress incontinence, the muscles preventing the leakage of urine have weakened. Any external pressures like a cough or a sneeze cause some of the urine to escape.

To treat this, we need to make the fingers stronger to hold the balloon closed. We can do this through exercise (pelvic floor muscle training) or by giving hormones (vaginal estrogen therapy). We can also add other things to help support the fingers such as tying a knot around the end of the balloon – this is analogous to a surgical option for treating stress incontinence.

Twin-to-Twin Transfusion Syndrome

An All-You-Can-Eat Buffet

There are many types of identical twins; some have separate placentas and amniotic sacs (room in which the baby lives), some share the placenta but have separate rooms and some share the placenta as well as the room. For those that share the placenta but are in separate rooms, it is important for doctors to be on the lookout for a condition called twin-to-twin transfusion syndrome. In this syndrome, the babies share a single food source; the placenta. The placenta is like an all-you-can-eat buffet provided by mum, providing the foetuses with all of their nutrients and oxygen. The only problem is that when two babies are sharing the buffet, one of the twins might be a bit greedy and take food from the other twin. In this case, the greedy baby will grow bigger with more fluid around them, while the other twin won't be able to grow as big because they will have reduced fluid around them. This could have harmful consequences for both twins if not identified and managed early in the pregnancy.

Urge Incontinence

A Short-Tempered Friend

We all have a friend who has a short temper. Think of your bladder as this friend. Even the smallest thing may set them off. Similarly, even small amounts of urine may urge your bladder to go. There are things that may make the friend's temper even worse: drinking too much alcohol or coffee, or if they are unwell. Similarly, these things can worsen your urge incontinence.

There are a few things we can do to fix their short temper. Firstly we need to fix their lifestyle by removing or lowering caffeine and alcohol. Then, we can try to control their temper through training exercises where they attempt to hold their temper for a few hours at a time. This is similar to bladder training exercises, where you need to try and resist the urge to go to the toilet. You can start by telling yourself not to go for one hour, then two hours, then three hours and so forth. The friend also needs to relax a little. Similarly, there are medications we can give to relax your bladder.

Index